Surgery for Pulmonary Mycobacterial Disease

Editor

JOHN D. MITCHELL

THORACIC SURGERY CLINICS

www.thoracic.theclinics.com

Consulting Editor
M. BLAIR MARSHALL

February 2019 • Volume 29 • Number 1

ELSEVIER

1600 John F. Kennedy Boulevard • Suite 1800 • Philadelphia, Pennsylvania, 19103-2899

http://www.thoracic.theclinics.com

THORACIC SURGERY CLINICS Volume 29, Number 1
February 2019 ISSN 1547-4127, ISBN-13: 978-0-323-65585-9

Editor: John Vassallo (j.vassallo@elsevier.com)
Developmental Editor: Laura Fisher

Thoracic Surgery Clinics (ISSN 1547-4127) is published quarterly by Elsevier Inc., 360 Park Avenue South, New York, NY 10010-1710. Months of publication are February, May, August, and November. Business and editorial offices: 1600 John F. Kennedy Boulevard, Suite 1800, Philadelphia, PA 19103-2899. Periodicals postage paid at New York, NY, and additional mailing offices. Subscription prices are $382.00 per year (US individuals), $585.00 per year (US institutions), $100.00 per year (US students), $460.00 per year (Canadian individuals), $757.00 per year (Canadian institutions), $225.00 per year (Canadian and international students), $475.00 per year (international individuals), and $757.00 per year (international institutions). Foreign air speed delivery is included in all Clinics' subscription prices. All prices are subject to change without notice. **POSTMASTER:** Send address changes to Thoracic Surgery Clinics, Elsevier Health Sciences Division, Subscription Customer Service, 3251 Riverport Lane, Maryland Heights, MO 63043. **Customer Service (orders, claims, online, change of address): Telephone: 1-800-654-2452 (U.S. and Canada); 314-447-8871 (outside U.S. and Canada). Fax: 314-447-8029. E-mail: journalscustomerservice-usa@elsevier.com (for print support); journalsonlinesupport-usa@elsevier.com (for online support).**

Reprints. For copies of 100 or more, of articles in this publication, please contact Commercial Rights Department, Elsevier Inc., 360 Park Avenue South, New York, NY 10010-1710. Tel: 212-633-3874; Fax: 212-633-3820; E-mail: reprints@elsevier.com.

Thoracic Surgery Clinics is covered in *MEDLINE/PubMed (Index Medicus), EMBASE/Excerpta Medica, Science Citation Index Expanded (SciSearch®), Journal Citation Reports/Science Edition,* and *Current Contents®/Clinical Medicine.*

Contributors

CONSULTING EDITOR

M. BLAIR MARSHALL, MD, FACS
Chief, Division of Thoracic Surgery, Associate
Professor, Department of Surgery,
Georgetown University Medical Center,
Georgetown University School of Medicine,
Washington, DC, USA

EDITOR

JOHN D. MITCHELL, MD
Courtenay C. and Lucy Patten Davis
Endowed Chair in Thoracic Surgery,
Professor and Chief, Section of General
Thoracic Surgery, Division of Cardiothoracic
Surgery, University of Colorado School
of Medicine, Aurora, Colorado,
USA

AUTHORS

ARMEN O. AVETISYAN, MD, PhD
St. Petersburg State Research Institute of
Phthisiopulmonology, Saint Petersburg,
Russian Federation

ROBERT W. BELKNAP, MD
Director, Denver Metro Tuberculosis Program,
Associate Professor of Medicine, Division of
Infectious Diseases, Denver Health and
Hospital Authority and the University of
Colorado Health Sciences Center, Aurora,
Colorado, USA

CHARLES L. DALEY, MD
Chief, Division of Mycobacterial and
Respiratory Infections, Professor of Medicine,
National Jewish Health, Denver, Colorado,
USA; University of Colorado, Aurora, Colorado,
USA

WENDI K. DRUMMOND, DO, MPH
Department of Medicine, National
Jewish Health, Denver, Colorado,
USA

IRINA G. FELKER, PhD
Endoscopy Department, Federal State
Budgetary Institution, Novosibirsk
Tuberculosis Research Institute, Ministry of
Health of the Russian Federation, Novosibirsk,
Russian Federation

DAVID E. GRIFFITH, MD
Professor of Medicine, Pulmonary and Critical
Care Medicine, The University of Texas Health
Science Center at Tyler, Tyler, Texas,
USA

NIKOLAY GRISCHENKO, MD, PhD
Surgical Department, Federal State
Budgetary Institution, Novosibirsk
Tuberculosis Research Institute, Ministry of
Health of the Russian Federation, Novosibirsk,
Russian Federation

JOHN I. HOGAN, MD
Clinical Fellow, Division of Infectious
Diseases, Massachusetts General Hospital,
Harvard Medical School, Boston,
Massachusetts, USA

ROCÍO M. HURTADO, MD, DTM&H
Associate Physician and Director,
Mycobacterial Diseases Center, Division of
Infectious Diseases, Massachusetts General
Hospital, Assistant Professor, Harvard Medical
School, Boston, Massachusetts, USA

SHANNON H. KASPERBAUER, MD
Department of Medicine, National Jewish
Health, Denver, Colorado, USA; University
of Colorado, Aurora, Colorado,
USA

DENIS V. KRASNOV, MD, PhD
Surgical Department, Federal State Budgetary
Institution, Novosibirsk Tuberculosis Research
Institute, Ministry of Health of the Russian
Federation, Tuberculosis Department,
Novosibirsk State Medical University, Faculty
of Professional Development and Professional
Retraining of Doctors, Novosibirsk, Russian
Federation

VLADIMIR A. KRASNOV, MD, PhD
Tuberculosis Department, Novosibirsk State
Medical University, Faculty of Professional
Development and Professional Retraining of
Doctors, Director of the Federal State
Budgetary Institution, Novosibirsk
Tuberculosis Research Institute, Ministry of
Health of the Russian Federation, Novosibirsk,
Russian Federation

GRIGORII G. KUDRIASHOV, MD
St. Petersburg State Research Institute of
Phthisiopulmonology, Saint Petersburg,
Russian Federation

STACEY L. MARTINIANO, MD
Assistant Professor of Pediatrics, Department
of Pediatrics, Children's Hospital Colorado,
University of Colorado Denver School of
Medicine, Aurora, Colorado, USA

JOHN D. MITCHELL, MD
Courtenay C. and Lucy Patten Davis Endowed
Chair in Thoracic Surgery, Professor and Chief,
Section of General Thoracic Surgery, Division
of Cardiothoracic Surgery, University of
Colorado School of Medicine, Aurora,
Colorado, USA

SANDRA B. NELSON, MD
Associate Physician and Director, Program in
Musculoskeletal Infections, Division of
Infectious Diseases, Massachusetts General
Hospital, Assistant Professor, Harvard Medical
School, Boston, Massachusetts, USA

JERRY A. NICK, MD
Professor, Department of Medicine, National
Jewish Health, Denver, Colorado; Department
of Medicine, University of Colorado Denver
School of Medicine, Aurora, Colorado, USA

YANA K. PETROVA, PhD
Surgical Department, Federal State Budgetary
Institution, Novosibirsk Tuberculosis Research
Institute, Ministry of Health of the Russian
Federation, Novosibirsk, Russian Federation

A. THOMAS PEZZELLA, MD
Founder/Director, International Children's
Heart Fund, Boca Raton, Florida, USA

JULIE V. PHILLEY, MD
Associate Professor of Medicine, Pulmonary
and Critical Care Medicine, The University of
Texas Health Science Center at Tyler, Tyler,
Texas, USA

SERGEY V. SKLUEV, PhD
Endoscopy Department, Federal State
Budgetary Institution, Novosibirsk
Tuberculosis Research Institute, Ministry of
Health of the Russian Federation, Treatment
Faculty, Tuberculosis Department, Novosibirsk
State Medical University, Novosibirsk, Russian
Federation

DMITRY A. SKVORTSOV, PhD
Surgical Department, Federal State Budgetary
Institution, Novosibirsk Tuberculosis Research
Institute, Ministry of Health of the Russian
Federation, Novosibirsk, Russian Federation

TANIA A. THOMAS, MD, MPH
Assistant Professor, Division of Infectious
Diseases and International Health, Department
of Medicine, University of Virginia,
Charlottesville, Virginia, USA

PIOTR K. YABLONSKII, MD, PhD
Professor, St. Petersburg State Research
Institute of Phthisiopulmonology, Dean of the
Medical Faculty, St. Petersburg State University,
Saint Petersburg, Russian Federation

Contents

Tuberculosis (TB) parallels the history of human development from the Stone Age to the present. TB continues to be in the top 10 causes of global human mortality over that period. This article highlights the history of pulmonary TB from the onset of human existence to the present. Despite its long history, TB was slowly identified as a major cause of disease, and defined causation and significant treatment strategies advances over the past 150 years. TB remains a major challenge for definitive global prevention and cure. This article gives a brief overview of the history of TB.

An estimated 1.7 billion (23%) of the world's population is infected with *Mycobacterium tuberculosis* leading to more than 10 million new tuberculosis (TB) cases each year. TB is one of the top 10 causes of death globally and is the leading cause of death from a single infectious disease agent. The World Health Organization's ambitious End TB Strategy aims to achieve a 95% reduction in TB deaths and 90% reduction in TB incidence rates by 2035.

Tuberculosis (TB) remains a common cause of infection and disease in much of the world. The majority of disease occurs from reactivation months or years after initial infection and most often involves the lungs. Sputum smears for acid-fast bacilli remain the initial diagnostic test but have limited sensitivity and specificity. Nucleic acid amplification tests are more sensitive and specific and can detect some mutations that cause drug resistance. Treatment of TB resistant to rifamycins alone or in combination with isoniazid and other drugs remains difficult and should be done in consultation with an expert in treating drug-resistant disease.

Surgery for tuberculosis is becoming more relevant today. This article discusses the main indications, contraindications, features of operations, and perioperative period. This information is useful for practicing surgeons and specialists in the treatment of pulmonary tuberculosis.

Special Articles

Although less common as causes of musculoskeletal infection than pyogenic bacteria, both Mycobacterium tuberculosis and nontuberculous mycobacteria can infect bones and joints. Although tuberculous arthritis and osteomyelitis have been recognized for millennia, infections caused by nontuberculous mycobacteria are being identified more often, likely because of a more susceptible host population and improvements in diagnostic capabilities. Despite advances in modern medicine, mycobacterial infections of the musculoskeletal system remain particularly challenging to diagnose and manage. This article discusses clinical manifestations of musculoskeletal infections caused by Mycobacterium tuberculosis and nontuberculous mycobacteria. Pathogenesis, unique risk factors, and diagnostic and therapeutic approaches are reviewed.

Nontuberculous mycobacteria (NTM) are important emerging cystic fibrosis (CF) pathogens, with estimates of prevalence ranging from 6% to 13%. Diagnosis of NTM disease in patients with CF is challenging, as the infection may remain indolent in some, without evidence of clinical consequence, whereas other patients suffer significant morbidity and mortality. Treatment requires prolonged periods of multiple drugs and varies depending on NTM species, resistance pattern, and extent of disease. The development of a disease-specific approach to the diagnosis and treatment of NTM infection in CF patients is a research priority, as a lifelong strategy is needed for this high-risk population.

Mycobacterium tuberculosis is the leading cause of death worldwide from a single bacterial pathogen. The World Health Organization estimates that annually 1 million children have tuberculosis (TB) disease and many more harbor a latent form. Accurate estimates are hindered by underrecognition and challenges in diagnosis. To date, an accurate diagnostic test to confirm TB in children does not exist. Treatment is lengthy but outcomes are generally favorable with timely initiation. With the End TB Strategy, there is an urgent need for improved diagnostics and treatment to prevent the unnecessary morbidity and mortality from TB in children.

THORACIC SURGERY CLINICS

SERIES OF RELATED INTEREST

Surgical Clinics
http://www.surgical.theclinics.com
Surgical Oncology Clinics
http://www.surgonc.theclinics.com
Advances in Surgery
http://www.advancessurgery.com

THE CLINICS ARE AVAILABLE ONLINE!
Access your subscription at:
www.theclinics.com

Preface
A Tale of Two Infections

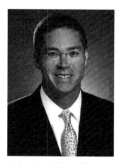

John D. Mitchell, MD

Editor

Borrowing from Charles Dickens, the current status of pulmonary mycobacterial disease, worldwide, is a tale of two infections. Certainly on a global scale, the main threat remains disease due to *Mycobacterium tuberculosis* (MTB), affecting approximately one-third of the world's population and over 9 million new cases annually. An increasing proportion of these individuals present with (or develop) drug-resistant tuberculosis, making medical treatment alone less effective. In 2016, the World Health Organization included, for the first time, recommendations regarding the selective use of surgery in the treatment of drug-resistant tuberculosis; the adjuvant use of surgery has been associated with improved cure rates in these difficult-to-treat cases.

In contrast, the recognition and treatment of pulmonary infection due to nontuberculous (atypical) mycobacteria (NTM) have lagged far behind those infected with standard *M* tuberculosis, although it is thought to be much more common in North America. NTM organisms are ubiquitous in the environment and do not cause infection through person-to-person contact, and thus are not reportable and tracked through standard public health mechanisms. As a result, the true incidence of NTM infection is unknown. In addition, the mechanisms of susceptibility remain obscure: why is it that some individuals contract infection, while their partners (seeing the same environmental exposures) remain healthy? Confusion in disease recognition and initiation of adequate treatment has led to increasing cases of significant drug resistance, which is incredibly difficult to overcome with medical therapy alone. As with MTB, the adjuvant use of surgical resection in selected NTM cases has been successful, although much more data are needed in this area.

Surgical treatment for pulmonary mycobacterial infection can be extremely challenging. Thoracic surgeons need to be familiar with all aspects of pulmonary mycobacterial disease and the indications for surgical intervention. The decision to employ adjuvant resection should be made in the multidisciplinary setting, where surgeons benefit greatly from the knowledge and input of their medical colleagues. In this issue, the medical and surgical treatment of both MTB and NTM pulmonary disease is discussed in detail, providing a worldwide perspective and guidance to all those who treat these difficult lung infections.

John D. Mitchell, MD
Section of General Thoracic Surgery
Division of Cardiothoracic Surgery
University of Colorado School of Medicine
C-310, Academic Office 1, Room 6607
12631 East 17th Avenue
Aurora, CO 80045, USA

E-mail address:
john.mitchell@ucdenver.edu

Thorac Surg Clin 29 (2019) ix
https://doi.org/10.1016/j.thorsurg.2018.10.001
1547-4127/19/© 2018 Published by Elsevier Inc.

History of Pulmonary Tuberculosis

A. Thomas Pezzella, MD

KEYWORDS

- Mycobacterium tuberculosis complex (MTBC) • TB- Tubercle bacillus • Sanatorium
- Collapse surgery • Thoracoplasty • Lung resection • Drug resistance • DOTS

KEY POINTS

- TB parallels human evolution and development.
- TB is preventive and curative with proper treatment and patient compliance.
- TB continues to be a major challenge in low-middle income countries and emerging economies.
- Expanded thoracic surgery role in TB treatment.

I KEEP six honest serving-men
(They taught me all I knew);
Their names are What and Why and When
And How and Where and Who.
I send them over land and sea,
I send them east and west;
But after they have worked for me,
I give them all a rest.

—Rudyard Kipling[1]

INTRODUCTION

Tuberculosis (TB) has been a major cause of illness and death in human society since antiquity. In 2016, one-fourth of the world population remained infected with TB. The annual incidence was 10.4 million, with an annual mortality rate of 1.3 million. Ten percent of the annual incidence, be it dormant, or latent, TB group will develop acute TB.[2] In contrast, in the United States in 2016, there were only 9287 new TB cases and a 2.9 in 100,000 case rate.[3]

The history of TB has been traced to the Stone Age Paleolithic period, circa 3.3 million years ago. It reached epidemic levels in Europe and North America in the eighteenth and nineteenth centuries. TB has decreased during the twentieth century in developed countries, but remains a serious threat in low-middle income countries (LMICs) and emerging economies (EEs), especially with the emergence of drug-resistant strains and the increasing association with human immunodeficiency virus (HIV). There have been a series of contemporary reviews of the history of TB.[4–13]

Thoracic surgery growth and development has its roots in the surgical care of patients with TB. The present review highlights the history of TB, encompassing the origin and history of TB, the continued prevalence of TB throughout the years, and the current role of medical treatment and thoracic surgery in the management of complex resistant TB in the twenty-first century.

BACKGROUND

It is important to understand the underlying social and economic aspects of human development. Epidemiologic transition serves as a basis to understand the evolution of diseases, especially TB. McKeown[14] highlights the epidemiologic transitions of Omran,[15] who identified 4 stages of human development: stage 1, the age of pestilence and famine; stage 2, the age of receding pandemics; stage 3, the age of degenerative and man-made diseases; and stage 4, the age of delayed degenerative diseases. However, Gersh and colleagues[16] have suggested a fifth stage that sees a rising epidemic with globally increasing

Disclosure: The author has nothing to disclose.
International Children's Heart Fund, 8378 Chisum Trail, Boca Raton, FL 33433, USA
E-mail address: atpezzella@hotmail.com

Thorac Surg Clin 29 (2019) 1–17
https://doi.org/10.1016/j.thorsurg.2018.09.002
1547-4127/19/© 2018 Elsevier Inc. All rights reserved.

noncommunicable disease that includes obesity, diabetes, and hypertension.

Svizzero and Tisdell[17] elaborated nicely on the Adam Smith theories of a sequential model age of human evolution. These stages included the 4 ages of hunters and gatherers, shepherds (pastoralism), agriculture, and commerce. The current age of commerce has created more socialization and human interaction, along with urbanization and the increased population growth and crowding, thus increasing the risk for disease transmission, especially for TB. TB has been involved in all the stages, either in a dormant or latent form, or an active form throughout the ages, yet has been more active and apparent during the periods of industrialization, migration, famine, poverty, and in areas of increased population density.

Globally, TB remains the ninth leading cause of global deaths, and the leading cause from a single infectious agent. In addition, in 2016, there were an additional 374,000 deaths among HIV-positive people. An estimated 10.4 million people fell ill with TB in 2016, and 56% of the total were living in 5 countries: India, Indonesia, China, Philippines, and Pakistan. Associated TB with HIV, as well as TB drug resistance remains a continuing threat and challenge. There were 600,000 new cases with resistance to rifampicin (RRTB), the most effective first-line drug, of which 490,000 were multidrug-resistant TB (MDR-TB), and almost half of these cases were in India, China, and Russia.[18–21]

Globally, the TB mortality rate is now falling at a 3% per year rate. TB incidence is also decreasing at a rate of 2% per year. Between 2005 and 2015 the total TB mortality rate decreased by 17.4%.The global goal by 2020 is to improve to 4% to 5% per year and 10%, respectively.[19,20]

The disability-adjusted life year (DALY) is a measure of overall disease burden, expressed as the number of years lost due to ill-health, disability, or early death.[21] In the communicable disease group TB DALYs ranked 13th as the leading cause of DALYs in 1990, 15th in 2005, and 18th in 2015.

TUBERCULOSIS PRIMER

TB is an obligate aerobic infectious bacterial organism (*Mycobacterium tuberculosis* or MTB).[22,23] The tubercle bacillus is a resistant infectious organism, in that it has a thick waxed cell wall that gives protection against external and host forces. Roy and Milton[24] stress that TB may be the only communicable disease that is initiated only through aerosols deposited in the distal lung. Pulmonary tuberculosis is the major target organ involved in 85% of the victims, as it is transmitted by inhaling the infected droplets that are airborne with sneezing, coughing, speaking, or spiting.

From the lungs, TB can spread to other parts of the body (extrapulmonary disease) via the hematogenous, lymphatic, or direct extension pathways. Infection occurs in the lung with alveolar contact, then spreads distally with an inflammatory reaction and formation of a Ghon focus that can be seen on radiographs, then can spread to regional nodes (Ghon complex), followed by the formation of a tuberculoma that can progress to an open or closed cavity with a fibrous rim around a pool of inner acellular liquefaction, caseous necrosis, and finally lung fibrosis, destruction.

Further resultant sequelae includes hemoptysis, cavities with aspergillomas, and empyema. Datta and colleagues,[25] in 2016, studied the oxygen transport of pulmonary TB granulomas to confirm that low oxygen levels in the granuloma can impair the host immune response, whereas the tubular bacillus can adapt and continue to persist in a hypoxic environment.

The activation of latent bacterial infection in 10% of the infected patients is slow, and it can remain dormant for many years. A suppressed host immune system from stress or other illnesses, especially HIV, can activate and accelerate the infective process. This is important because it may explain the long-term ability of TB to survive in the human host.

Despite increased availability of medical treatment, new challenges have developed with the growing incidences of drug-resistant tuberculosis that include DR-TB (drug resistant), MDR-TB (multidrug resistant), XDR-TB (extensively drug resistant), XXDR-TB (extremely drug resistant), and TDR-TB (totally drug resistant). Social issues that enhance TB include poverty, poor education, migration, and urbanization with resultant crowding, pollution, and poor sanitation. No age group, country, or geographic location has been spared exposure to TB. Presently, with proper identification and management, TB is diagnosable, preventable, controllable, and curative.

EARLY HISTORY

The origin and history of TB follows 4 time lines that include the following: (1) the early or ancient archeological findings, along with modern scientific DNA methodology testing; (2) documentation from the medical and nonmedical literature and events; (3) the discovery of the causation of TB; and (4) the subsequent treatment modalities of TB. The latter time lines can be further divided into 5 parts: folk care and medicinal offerings, sanatoriums, thoracic surgery, medical drugs, and emerging strategies for combined medical and adjuvant surgical approaches.[26–35]

The earlier aspects and evolution of TB have been well studied and recorded. Archeological and paleontological discoveries and evidence of decayed human or animal teeth or bones, especially the vertebral bones (Pott disease) in Egyptian mummy structures, have traditionally been the major source of TB identification.[5] This has been supported and supplemented by modern scientific molecular genotyping (ancient DNA [aDNA], modern DNA [mDNA]), DNA sequencing with single nucleotide polymorphisms, and polymerase chain reaction testing (**Box 1**).[26–29] Presently, there are refined genotyping methods to study the *M tuberculosis* strains.[30–35] The path of TB from East Africa accompanied the migration of *Homo sapiens* to the rest of the world, especially along the established trade routes with increased mingling and crowding of populations (**Fig. 1**).[30]

An accurate or definitive history of the origin, evolution, and spread of the *M tuberculosis* complex (MTBC) genus/species that includes *M tuberculosis*, *Mycobacterium bovis*, *Mycobacterium microti*, *Mycobacterium africanum*, *Mycobacterium pinnipedii*, *Mycobacterium caprae*, and *Mycobacterium canetti* species, remain and continue to evolve.

As noted, TB has been known to mankind since ancient times. It has been postulated that TB has existed for at least 150 million years.[5] Gutierrez and colleagues,[31] in 2005, postulated that MTBC was the clonal progeny of a single progenitor ancestor (*Mycobacterium prototuberculosis*) that dated back more than 3 million years, and started in East Africa where early hominids were located.

This progeny occurred from an evolutionary bottleneck that occurred 20,000 to 35,000 years ago. With migration out of East Africa starting

approximately 10,000 years ago, MTBC underwent changes or lineages, along with the development of agriculture and domestication, and the resultant changes or adjustments in the host human mDNA. This has been supported by molecular aDNA and mDNA testing.[32–34] Gagneux,[30] in 2016, confirmed that MTBC is an ancient disease that evolved with humanity and not animals in East Africa, with humans as the primary host. It developed the ability to remain dormant and reemerge many years later. TB diversity increased as the human population increased during the migratory phase out of East Africa. At the same time, Gagneux[30] postulated that humans may have developed increased immunity to TB. This makes a case for host-pathogen coevolution. This is defined as "reciprocal, adaptive genetic changes in interacting host and pathogen species."[30] **Box 1** highlights several historical global fossils, in humans or animals. Namouchi and colleagues[35] support the theory that TB is a successful pathogen that emerged from the bottleneck with the ability to diversify by recombination and natural selection.

FOLK LORE, FOLK REMEDIES, MYTHS, AND SCIENCE

There is a paucity of credible documented scientific literature sources regarding the discovery and description of TB during the ancient period, Middle Ages, and Renaissance that has given factual insight into the causation or natural history of TB.[4–13] Fear and acceptance dominated this time frame. The recorded literature concentrated on the bizarre and lethal occurrences that affected all levels of society.[36] The time line of activity is divided into the BC and AD periods.[37]

Boxes 2 and **3**[38–40] highlight the documented sources of those time periods. Once the existence of TB was suspected, discovered, or appreciated, then a series of medical and nonmedical writings, terms, observations, and theories evolved during the latter ancient period, and extended through the Middle Ages, the Renaissance, and the modern period. Most of these iterations were stroked by the fears, misery, and romanticizing of this strange and lethal phenomenon, along with a plethora of ineffective therapeutic remedies, and futile attempts to explore, define, or understand the TB causation.

Many lingering disagreements and debates centered around hereditary and acquired contagion causation. Prevailing medical evaluation and treatment cures were still influenced by the Hippocrates and Galen humors theories.[39] Both believed that TB (phthisis) was the most widespread of all

---

Box 1
Ancient time line human and animal tuberculosis (TB) identification

- United States: Bison: 17,000 years ago: ancient DNA (aDNA)[26]
- Israel: Alit-Yam: Neolithic period: 9000 years ago: woman and child aDNA[27]
- Germany: 5450 to 4780 BC: aDNA[28]
- Egypt: Mummies: 2400 BC: Pott's lesions with degenerative tubercular lesions on the thoracic spine
- Peru: Paracas-Caverna women, 1001 to 1300 AD: aDNA[29]

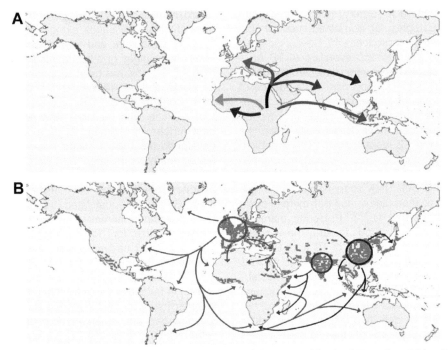

Fig. 1. Out-of-and-back-to-Africa. The evolutionary history of the out and back of TB to East Africa. MTBC originated in East Africa and some lineages accompanied the out and back Africa migrations of modern humans. The evolutionary modern MTBC lineages spread, and expanded with increases in human populations throughout the global regions (each *dark gray dot* corresponds to 1 million people) via exploration, trade, and conquest. In (*A*) the 3 colors represent the three evolutionary lineages. (*From* Hershberg R, Lipatov M, Small PM, et al. High functional diversity in *Mycobacterium tuberculosis* driven by genetic drift and human demography. PLoS Biol 2008;6(12):e311; with permission.)

the diseases of that time. Hippocrates believed that tuberculosis was hereditary, whereas Galen believed the disease was essentially contagious.[39]

Aretaeus of Cappadocia[40] defined the cause of the disease in which phthisis was a pulmonary abscess that produced cough, fever, increased expectoration, and emaciation.

A number of terms reflected the effects of TB. Consumption was the translation of a Sanskrit word (1000 BC) for a wasting disease. Hippocrates coined the word phthisis (decaying) to describe the disease. Scars from TB cervical lymph nodes were called scrofula (**Fig. 2**). They were called "Kings Evil" by the king, and it was widely believed that the kings of England and France could cure scrofula by touching those affected, as well as relieving symptoms like hacking cough, bloody cough, miasmas, and fatigue. A number of other terms have been recorded that defined or characterized the TB atm during those turbulent times (**Box 4**).[41]

A mystical culture, along with folklore also surrounded TB. A notable example was vampirism:

When people died from consumption and other members of their household soon sickened as well, it was believed that the dead family member was visiting the house at night as a vampire and slowly sucking their lives away. Because tuberculosis patients were slowly being "consumed" by the disease, it was assumed that vampires were feeding off of their blood.[42]

Another example of folk theory was advanced in 1530 by Paracelsus. He believed that tuberculosis was caused by a failure of an internal organ to accomplish its alchemical duties. When this occurred in the lungs, stony precipitates would develop causing tuberculosis in what he called the tartaric process.[43]

Folk remedies were widespread. Galen recommended fresh air, human breast milk, wolf livers, and phlebotomy, as well as diet, exercise for children, rest for adults, and sunlight (ultraviolet light or heliotherapy).

A bevy of preventive methods with plausible effects included the following: no spitting, the use of spittoons (pinger was the sound of wet tobacco when it hit the spittoon); house cleaning with antiseptic carbolic acid; avoiding women's trailing skirts; and not sweeping dry floors, thus avoiding contaminated dust inhalation. Other preventive or palliative measures without proven efficacy

Box 2
BC documented time line sources

- Old Testament: (3700–3300 BC): Leviticus 26:16 and Deuteronomy 28:22, the Lord threatened his people with a plague; this plague was called "consumption."[38]
- The Code of Hammurabi: Babylonian law code (circa 1754 BC).
- India (1500 BC): Vedas/Rigveda.
- Middle East: Clay tablets from library of Assyrian King Assurbanipal (668–626 BC).
- Herodotus (484–425 BC) "Histories."
- Hippocrates (460–375 BC): Phthisis (decaying); Aphorisms, Book 1 "Of the Epidemics"; believed TB was hereditary.[39]
- China: Huang TiNei-Ching (Chinese Medical Journal) 400 BC.
- Aretaeus of Cappadocia (200 BC) in Chapter VIII of his *First Book on Chronic Diseases*, formed the most accurate descriptions of diseases, especially pulmonary TB symptoms.[40]
- Galen of Pergamon (131–201) suspected the contagious nature of phthisis, in deference to the hereditary theory of the disease. He warned against contact with consumptives, and recommended a treatment plan of fresh air, rest, and nutrition. This thinking continued for many years thereafter.

included foods like plantain, nuts, honey, and pomegranates; cod liver oil; and medicinals, like hyssop, eucalyptus, opioids, and moxibustion-mugwort burned on the skin.

During the eighteenth and nineteenth centuries, the tuberculosis debate between hereditary versus contagious causation continued. By the end of the nineteenth century, with the increasing population growth in urban areas, 70% to 90% of the populations of Europe and North America were infected with TB, and more than 80% of those with active tuberculosis died.[44] In Europe, the annual mortality rate for TB was 800 to 1000 per 100,000 people.[6]

These tragic events were highlighted and witnessed by many prominent individuals that included poets, writers, artists, rulers, and philosophers who suffered and died from TB during that period (**Box 5**). The poorly ventilated and congested urban dwellings, along with primitive sanitation, hygiene, and poverty, all contributed to the increased TB morbidity and mortality. In addition, increasing migration, expanding trade routes, and the onset of the industrial revolution prolonged the phenomenon of this great white plague. Other

concentrated areas for increased TB activity included hospitals, shelters, and prisons.

The feelings of the victims were expressed in their writings and works. Ralph Waldo Emerson, the American essayist called his consumptive partner "too lovely to live long." The paintings of Dante Gabriel Rossetti were filled with pale, thin girls with their hair cascading over their shoulders. Even now, in the late twentieth century, the singer Van Morrison dedicated a beautiful song, "TB Sheets" to a dying friend.[45]

In the early twentieth century, notable thoracic surgeons were also infected with TB. Examples included Edward Archibald and Norman Bethune from Canada; and John Alexander and Alfred Blalock from the United States. Not surprisingly, they all played an active role in developing TB surgical procedures, even as they dealt with their own TB illness.

Specific scientific progress slowly evolved over the ensuing years, especially in Europe.

In 1546, Hieronymus Fracastorius described contagion theory. This increased the search for the cause and spread of this dreadful illness.

In 1679, Franciscus Sylvius described the progress of the disease in his *Opera Medica*. Using chemical principles, he highlighted the TB nodules as tubercula.

In 1790, Benjamin Martin believed the disease was caused by heredity but was possibly acquired and infectious.

In 1720, Benjamin Martin, in *A New Theory of Consumption*, hypothesized that TB resulted from the actions of "wonderfully minute living creatures." Once established in the body, they would generate the symptoms of consumption.

In 1816, Rene Theophile Laennec invented the stethoscope, as well as increasing the understanding of the pathogenesis of TB in *Traite du Diagnostic des Maladies*. He studied the pathogenesis of tuberculosis in detail. In 1819, he combined the pulmonary and extrapulmonary manifestations of TB into one common understanding and pathway. This improved the diagnostic capability.

In 1839, Johann Lucas Schönlein declared the TB tubercle was the basis of the disease.

In 1865, Jeon-Antoine Villemin showed that TB was both infectious and transmittable; that is, a contagion. He demonstrated that one could infect a healthy rabbit with tuberculosis from infected cadaver tissue. This was a major breakthrough, because medical theory at that time held that each case of consumption arose spontaneously in predisposed people.

In 1882, there occurred a sentinel event. Robert Koch used a new staining method of the sputum

Box 3
AD time line sources

- Pliny the Younger: 71. Letter to Priscus: Letters V11.
- Clarissimus Galen (129–200): contagion, blood-letting to cure.
- Avicenna: 1020 AD. The Canon of Medicine. Recognized TB as a contagious infectious disease. He also developed the quarantine concept to limit the spread of TB through contact with soil and water.
- Girolamo Hieronymus Fracastorius: 1546. De Morbis Contagiosis. Declared TB as contagious.
- Paracelsus: 1530: internal organs were unable to do alchemical duties.[43]
- Franciscus Sylvius: 1679: specified phthisis, and its relationship with the lungs. His work De Contagione postulated that phthisis was transmitted by an invisible virus.
- Richard Morton (1637–1698): described a relationship among glands, tubercles, and consumption of the lungs.
- Benjamin Martel: 1720: developed theory for Consumption.
- E. Barry: 1726: drained purulent TB lung cavity.
- Matthew Baillie: 1793: caseous necrosis and abscesses were named tubercles.
- Gaspard Bayle: 1810: described disseminated miliary TB.
- Leopold Auenbrugger: 1808: clinical chest percussion methods.[49]
- Rene Theophile Laennec: 1819: D'Auscultation Mediate: unified pathologies of lung and lesions within the body. Claimed that the tubercle must be present in phthisis. Invented the stethoscope method of inspection.
- James Carson: 1819: initiated the concept of collapse therapy.
  - J. L. Schönlein: 1839: attributed with naming the disease, tuberculosis, rather than consumption, because tubercle was basis of the disease.
  - Hermann Brehmer: 1859: sanatorium pioneer.
  - Pasteur: 1860s: described airborne transmission, and germ theory.
  - Jean-Antoine Villemin: 1865 AD: Cause et nature de la tuberculos: son inculpation de l'homme au lapin. Inoculated rabbits with TB fluid from dead TB victim and rabbit remained alive, but at autopsy 3 months later TB was found. Confirmed TB was contagious.
  - Robert Koch: 1882 AD: TB presentation "Die Aetiologie der Tuberculosis" confirmed isolated of tubercle bacilli:
    - Used new technology (microscope).
    - Invented a method to prove causation (Koch's postulates).[45]
    - Lesion is secondary to infection by a germ that is tubercle bacillus; in 1890 developed a glycerine extract of the tubercle bacilli as a remedy for tuberculosis called tuberculin. It was not effective, but was later adapted as a test for asymptomatic tuberculosis.
- Albert Calmette and Camilo Guerin: 1908: developed a TB vaccine from attenuated bovine-strain tuberculosis. It was called BCG (Bacillus of Calmette and Guerin). It was first tested on humans in 1921 but was not used until after World War II.
- In 1908, a tuberculin sensitivity screening skin test was developed (purified protein derivative or Mantoux test) by Mendel and Mantoux.[50]
- The Ziehl-Neelsen stain or acid-fast stain, described by Franz Ziehl (1859–1926) and Friedrich Neelsen (1854–1898).
- 1854: Hermann Brehmer established the first German sanatorium for the systematic open-air treatment of tuberculosis.
- William Wells and colleagues in the1950s: confirmed airborne TB transmission.
- Selman Waksman, Albert Schatz, Elizabeth Bugia:1944: discovery of streptomycin.
- Jörgen Lehmann:1944: develops antibiotic 4-aminosalicylic acid (PAS).
- E.H. Robitzek and I.J. Selikoff: 1952: discovery of isoniazid, then ethambutol in 1962.

- Once isoniazid became available, attention turned to the drugs needed in combination to avoid the development of resistance. Triple therapy of isoniazid, streptomycin, and PAS became the standard triple therapy until the availability of rifampin in 1966.
- 1995: The World Health Organization launches DOTS (Directly Observed Treatment, Short-Course) program as a control strategy for tuberculosis.

Data from Refs.[4–13]

from TB patients. This established *M tuberculosis* bacteria (tubercle bacillus) as the etiology and cause of the clinical disease (**Fig. 3**). The Ziehl-Neelsen microscopic acid-fast stain was described by the bacteriologist Franz Ziehl (1859–1926) and the pathologist Friedrich Neelsen (1854–1898). Using the microscope, Koch showed that the thick cover of the organism's protein made it difficult to visualize unless a specific spot of oxide of the Zeihl-Neelson oxide stain was removed. The bacteria were termed the Koch bacillus and because it took red acid dye, the red rods were called acid-fast bacilli or red snappers. Later investigations proved that air and secretions expelled from consumptive lungs contained live bacteria. These were the defining moments in the history of TB. Koch was awarded the Nobel Prize in 1905 for this seminal accomplishment.[46]

The Koch Postulates demonstrated the relationship between agent and disease[47]. Koch also developed a glycerine extract of the tubercle bacilli as a remedy for tuberculosis in 1890, calling it "tuberculin," yet it was not effective, especially for children, and was terminated.

In 1895, Wilhelm Konrad Roentgen developed the radiograph, which advanced the diagnoses of TB. The chest radiograph became a standard diagnostic tool that revealed the tubercular pulmonary lesions, even before any clinical symptoms had developed. However, because the pictures did not distinguish between healed and dormant lesions, a bacterial test was needed to supplement and confirm the diagnosis.[48] This was resolved in 1908 when a tuberculin sensitivity screening skin test was developed (PPD or purified protein derivative or Mantoux test) by Mendel and Mantoux.[49]

In addition, bedside clinical teaching was initiated by Pierre-Joseph Desault in the late eighteenth century. Joseph Leopold Auenbrugger introduced chest percussion in the early nineteenth century, along with Dr Rene Laennec's invention of the stethoscope.[50]

These events heralded a major turning point or paradigm shift in the understanding and approach to TB diagnosis and treatment. This now provided a more complete pathway to accurately complete the assessment and diagnosis of the unfortunate TB victims.

TREATMENT EVOLUTION
Sanatorium

It was clear that the lists of treatments during the previous centuries were of questionable effect, in terms of specific prevention or cure.[13] As noted,

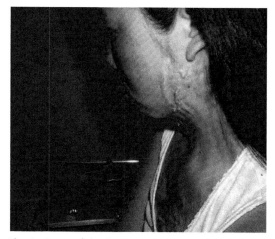

Fig. 2. TB scrofula. (*Courtesy of* A. Thomas Pezzella, MD, Boca Raton, FL.)

Box 4
Examples of descriptive phrases for TB

Phthisis (Greek for decaying)

Consumption (to eat up or devour)

Lupus vulgaris (TB of the skin)

Pott's TB disease of vertebral bodies

Captain of all of these men

Grave yard cough

The robber of youth

Great white plague

White Death

Grave yard cough

King's Evil

Contagion

Lactic fever

Gastric fever

Box 5
Sampling of famous historical victims of TB

St Francis Assisi (1226) Italian Catholic priest

Honore de Balzac (1799–1850), French writer

Anne Bronte (1816–1849), English writer

Emily Bronte (1818–1848), English writer

Elizabeth Barrett Browning (1806–1861), English writer

Anton Chekhov (1860–1904), Russian writer

Frederic Chopin (1810–1849), French composer

Stephen Crane (1871–1900), American writer

Franz Kafka (1883–1924), German writer

John Keats (1795–1821), English poet

Vivian Leigh (1913–1967), English actress

Louis XIII, (1601–1643), King of France

Louis XVII (1785–1795), King of France

Katherine Mansfield (1888–1923), New Zealand writer

George Orwell (1903–1950), English writer

Robert Louis Stevenson (1850–1894), Scottish writer

Henry David Thoreau (1817–1862), American writer

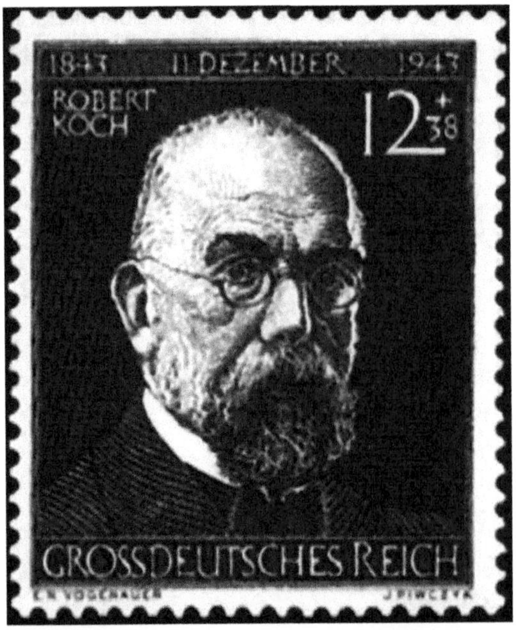

Fig. 3. Robert Koch stamp, 1843. (*From* Shampo MA, Rosenow EC. A history of tuberculosis on stamps. Chest 2009;136:580; with permission.)

the clinical diagnosis of TB had improved based on the objective data that included clinical suspicion, history, and physical examination, especially chest percussion and the stethoscope, skin testing with PPD (+after 3–10 weeks-latent TB), positive sputum acid-fast stain (Ziehl-Neelsen) with greater than 100 red snappers per high-powered field (HPF), or the auramine-rhodamine stain (AR) fluorescence microscopy, that displayed a reddish-yellow fluorescence. A positive Lowenstein-Jenson medium culture was developed in 1932,[51] and, along with the chest radiograph, completed the evaluation.

This allowed earlier definitive recognition, diagnosis, and subsequent isolation of both asymptomatic and symptomatic infected individuals, be it voluntary or involuntary confinement or incarceration in the sanatorium. The laws or regulations, regarding voluntary or nonvoluntary quarantine or confinement to home, hospital, or sanatorium, have varied over time in most countries.[52] This became a controversial subject with regard to personal rights and public health protection, and continues to the present.

The concept of a TB sanatorium arose with isolation and possible cure of TB in places that provided a protected and secure environment. The patients were isolated from family and society, and treated with fresh air, sunlight exposer, rest, relaxation, improved nutrition, and proper sanitation and hygiene.

The first sanatorium was initiated in 1859 by Hermann Brehmer, in Gobersdorf, Germany.[53] In the United States, the first sanatorium was started in 1875 by Joseph Gleitsmann in Asheville, North Carolina. In 1886, Edward Livingston Trudeau founded the Adirondack Cottage sanatorium at Saranac Lake, New York.[54]

Fitzsimons General Hospital #21, in Denver, Colorado was established in 1918 for returning World War I soldiers with TB.[55] Clustered soldiers in the damp dirty trenches created a high-risk atmosphere for TB infection, and TB was a major cause for discharge following the war.[7]

In Europe, the largest TB sanatorium (3500 beds) from 1932 to 1940 was established at Eugenio Morelli Hospital in Sondalo, Italy.[56] The results of the sanatorium experience are difficult to accurately document insofar as symptom relief and curative effect. The psychological relief, along with fresh air, a relaxed environment, and balanced nutrition had a salutary effect, along with an enhanced immunologic boost. Varying types of sequestered facilities also evolved. The overall results of the sanatorium era are not clear. The death rate in sanatoriums or at home were the same. Approximately half of patients died whether they were treated in a sanatorium or treated at home.[57]

Daniel[5] noted a report from 1923 in which the results of 4000 patients with 5-year follow-up were studied. Fourteen percent of sanatorium sputum-negative patients died, whereas 38% of home-treated patients died. For sputum-positive patients, the split was 61% and 81% mortality.

In summary, the sanatorium experience was a mixed physical and psychological experience for most, and unlike the spiritual malaise as experienced by Hans Castorp in *The Magic Mountain* novel by Thomas Mann.[58]

Thoracic Tuberculin Surgery

Stop at the pleura

— *Ernest Dieffenback*[59]

The history of TB surgery has been well reviewed.[59–64]

Thoracic surgery advanced with the discovery of the radiograph in 1895. This allowed an anatomic view of the TB pathology within the chest cavity. Then the development, and severity of TB could be objectively evaluated. However, thoracic surgery at the end of the nineteenth century was somewhat limited because surgical entry to the chest cavity beyond the chest pleura was not advised or advocated for fear that opening the pleura would compromise the patient's negative lung pressure. This changed with the advances in anesthesia and positive airway control and management.

The time line for TB surgery is summarized in (**Box 6**). It is ironic that the goal changed from external fresh air to the lungs in the sanatorium era to relaxing the lung and suppressing oxygen entry with surgical collapse and resection techniques. Both the sanatorium and surgery approach complemented each other in the early stages, because many sanatorium patients went on to have surgery with increasing successful outcomes.

In 1821, the concept of collapse was originally advanced by Dr James Carson. There was a long lapse before the collapse concept was further developed. Collapse surgery with the artificial pneumothorax procedure, using a pneumothorax apparatus, was initiated by Carlo Forlanini in 1882.[65] The rationale was that the affected lung would collapse, thus allowing the lung to "rest" and heal. However, the pneumothorax was limited to the upper lung TB cavities, yet it remained popular for many years.[56]

The procedure involved inserting a long needle between the patient's ribs and pumping the chest cavity with filtered air to a goal of zero pressure in the created space. This allowed the diseased lung to rest, because the lung could not heal under the constant irritation of inflation and deflation.[66] This technique required "multiple refills" over several years. In addition, incomplete collapse, secondary to residual adhesions, restricted total collapse.[56]

Jacobaeus, in 1912, introduced the thorascopic closed intrapleural pneumolysis procedure utilizing a galvanocautery.[64,67,68] This was the early forerunner of the current video-assisted thoracoscopic surgery procedure that decreased the blind finger method. This approach was well received because it was less invasive and more effective in patients in whom adhesions prevented a satisfactory result by the open technique.

As noted, artificial pneumothorax was used primarily in patients with TB cavitary disease. It was postulated that collapse would limit disease spread by inducing fibrosis and encapsulation of the infected area. More likely, by impairing ventilation to the treated lung, and collapsing the cavity within, it reduced oxygen levels and inhibited growth of the oxygen-dependent tubercle bacillus.

Because air injected during pneumothorax therapy was resorbed after 1 to 2 weeks, recurrent injections were required (usually repeated over 1–2 years). The risk of pleuritis often prevented maintenance of the collapse. Other complications included infection and bleeding into the pleural space.

Further advances with collapse therapy continued, as these early approaches were not very effective over the long term, especially with lower lung and bilateral cavities. For lower-lobe cavities, other less invasive methods were performed. Pneumoperitoneum, in which air was injected into the abdominal cavity, resulting in diaphragmatic elevation or, with phrenic nerve crush, where the diaphragm it innervated was temporarily paralyzed, were both marginally effective, but not difficult to perform, and often used together.[69]

Thoracoplasty was a major advance in TB surgery.[60–62] In 1885, Edouard Bernard de Cerenville introduced the thoracoplasty procedure for apical cavitary disease. In 1922, Ludolf Brauer and Paul Friedrich developed a more radical thoracoplasty involving 2 to 9 ribs. These procedures were performed under local anesthesia with high mortality. In 1912, Ernst Sauerbruch and Max Wilms developed a less radical thoracoplasty that involved primarily the extrapleural paravertebral ribs and the transverse processes.

Thoracoplasty was developed to induce long-term collapse, but it was an extensive and mutilating procedure. This operation carried

---

Box 6
Timeline of TB surgery

Giorgio Baglivi: 1696: improvement of TB patient following pneumothorax injury from chest sword wound

F.H. Ramge:1834: successful therapeutic pneumothorax

James Carson: 1819: initiated the concept of collapse

Carlo Forlanini: 1882: artificial pneumothorax[65]

J. Hastings and R. Storks: 1844: cavernostomy

Crawford Long: 1842: Ether gas applied anesthesia

William Morton: 1846: discovery of anesthesia

John Collins Warren: first operation with anesthesia at the Ether dome in Massachusetts General Hospital, Boston, Massachusetts

Edouard Bernard de Cerenville: 1885: Costal resection (2–4 ribs)

Anesthesia: 1882: open drop method with either or chloroform and spontaneous negative breathing

Carl Spengler: 1890: successful apicolysis with extrapleural plombage procedure

Theodore Tuffier: 1891: first partial lung resection (apicolysis): the forerunner of the extrapleural plombage; 1896: with cuffed endotracheal tube

Joseph O'Dwyer/George Fell: 1888: invented the respirator apparatus

E. Delorme: 1894: decortication

Rudolph Matas:1898: performed chest wall surgery with Fell device

Wilhelm Conrad Roentgen: 1895: invention of radiograph

Brauer/Friedrich: 1929: thoracoplasty with first rib left intact

Hans Christian Jacobaeus: 1912: thorascopic closed intrapleural pneumolysis of pleural adhesions

Ernst Sauerbruch/Wilm: 1912: paravertebral thoracoplasty; inventor of the negative-pressure chamber

Samuel Meltzer and John Auer: 1904: anesthesia via endotracheal access and positive-pressure ventilation

H. Schlange: 1907: extrapleural plombage

A. Stuertz: 1912: phrenicectomy

A. Bernou: 1922: plombage with oleothorax (vegetable and mineral oil) (see **Fig. 5**)

Leo Eloesser: 1924: division of adhesions extrapleurally to avoid lung tears; developed open drainage technique[79] (see **Fig. 6**)

Harold Brunn: 1929: 1-stage lobectomy with individual ligation of hilar vessels and suture of bronchial stump

Heidenhain Lilienthal: 1933: first successful pneumonectomy for TB mass hilar ligation

Samuel Freedlander: 1934: successfully excised the right upper lobe of a patient with a tuberculous cavity who had failed collapse therapy

Carl Semb: 1935: apicolysis via subperiosteal approach

John Alexander: 1934: major thoracoplasty pioneer; also performed thoracic muscle plombage (Alexander J. Supraperiosteal and subcostal pneumolysis with filling of pectoral muscle. Arch Surg 1934;28:538–547)

Vincent Monaldi: 1939: cavernostomy (2-stage intracavitary aspiration)

Churchill/Klopstock: 1943: lobectomy with individual vessel ligation technique

---

considerable morbidity and mortality. As a consequence, it was often performed in 2 or 3 stages at 2-week to 3-week intervals to allow gradual realignment of the mediastinum. The operation involved disarticulation of the ribs with preservation of the costal periosteum, so that with time the rib would regenerate into a position inducing permanent pulmonary collapse. The ultimate goal was to reduce or decrease the thoracic cage volume, thus allowing collapse of the cavity and obliteration of the extrapleural space.

A variety of thoracoplasty techniques emerged (**Boxes 7** and **8**). John Alexander is credited with refining the thoracoplasty approaches to surgical collapse therapy with his 2 seminal publications in 1925 and 1937.[62,70,71] Langston[72] gave a very

---

Box 7
Other TB surgical methods or procedures of historical interest

Sandbag or diseased side down

Intrapleural pneumonolysis with apicolysis (injection of sterile air, or paraffin)

Pneumoperitoneum

Multiple intercostal neurectomy (decreases costal excursions)

Scalenotomy (divide) or scalenectomy (excise) (decreases upper costal excursions and depresses the lung apex)

Phrenic nerve crush or paralysis with/without transection of accessory muscle

Extrapleural plombage or pneumothorax (space between parietal pleura and endothoracic fascia)[74] (see **Fig. 4**).

Subcostal and extraperiosteal plombage ("bird cage") (periosteum stripped from upper 5 ribs) (Lucite balls most commonly used)

Pulmonary artery ligation (Sauerbruch/ Schlaepfer)

Types of thoracoplasty techniques:

Simon: 1869: thoracoplasty for empyema

J.A. Estlander: 1879: decostalization of chest wall

Schede: 1890: resection of ribs, intercostals muscles, and pleural peel

Alexander: 1928: Staged thoracoplasty (usually 3) sessions

Grow: 1946: excision of parietal peel

Kergin: 1953: excision of thick parietal peel

Bjork: 1954: osteoplastic thoracoplasty in 1 stage maintains chest wall stability

Tailored (modified): 1959: tailoring the thoracoplasty (number of ribs) to size of resectional spine; done 3 to 4 weeks before lung resection

Andrews: 1961: thoracomediastinal plication

Eloesser flap: 1935[79]

Cavernostomy: Monaldi[80]

Box 8
Changes in most common TB operations

Procedures in 1943:

  Phrenic paralysis

  Pneumothorax

    Intrapleural pneumonolysis

  Pneumoperitoneum

  Thoracoplasty

  Cavernostomy

  Pulmonary resection

Procedures in 1968:

  Pulmonary resection

  Thoracoplasty

    Standard

    Plombage

  Cavernostomy

From Steele JD. The surgical treatment of pulmonary tuberculosis. Ann Thorac Surg 1968;6:485; with permission.

---

scholarly overview of the evolutionary steps that led from the early primitive Schede thoracoplasty to the Alexander version.

Because of the complexity and complications associated with thoracoplasty, extraperiosteal, and extrapleural plombage evolved. Plombage could be performed as a single localized procedure and did not cause respiratory paradox or major mediastinal shifts in the postoperative period. Because lung function was preserved, it could be used in patients with more limited cardiopulmonary reserve or comorbidity.

Plombage was performed by dissecting the costal periosteum and intercostal muscles off the ribs to create an extrapleural space. A variety of materials were used to fill the space and collapse the underlying TB cavity. These fillers included fat (omentum, fresh lipoma), paraffin, wax, silk, gelatin, bone, gauze sponge, rubber balloons, methyl-methacrylate (Lucite balls), as well as vegetable and mineral oil (Oleothorax).[73]

Several complications occurred with this technique, including infection, migration of the materials, and erosion of blood vessels. It was initially recommended that the fillers be removed at 6 to 12 months to avoid these complications,[69] but were not always adhered to. This procedure may be particularly attractive for high-risk patients. This technique is still performed in some centers[74] (**Fig. 4**).

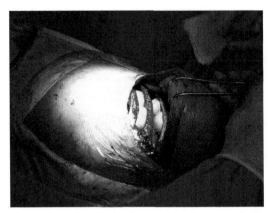

Fig. 4. Extrapleural plombage with ping pong balls. (*Courtesy of* A. Thomas Pezzella, MD, Boca Raton, FL.)

Resectional TB surgery evolution from thoracoplasty was not an uneventful transition.[61,62] Although attempted by Block in 1883, Tuffier successfully performed resection or apicolysis for TB in 1891. He used chloroform anesthesia and a second intercostal space approach, and the patient recovered without complications.[75] However, enthusiasm for resectional surgery did not increase until Friedlander's report in 1935. Despite the stiff cautions by Dr John Alexander who was a staunch supporter of thoracoplasty, resectional surgery advanced. Naef[63] nicely highlights the initial Shenstone hilar tourniquet technique that was used for the lobectomy. Harold Brunn, in 1929, developed the mass-suture ligation. Howard Lilienthal pioneered the resection technique in 1910, with a 2-stage approach that ligated the lobe, and allowed it to slough out the open wound. From 1914 he adopted the 1-stage resection and his 1922 report of 30 cases using the tourniquet had an overall 43% mortality. By 1940, mortality had decreased to 20.5% in the combined experiences of surgeons.[61,62]

The anesthesia techniques used during the late nineteenth century period consisted of local anesthesia with spontaneous patient breathing that allowed coughing and expirations that could cause lung contamination, or open drop anesthesia with ether or chloroform and spontaneous breathing.[59]

In 1904, Ferdinand Sauerbruch introduced low-pressure ventilation in an open chest that was maintained with the patient in a negative-pressure chamber.[62] Subsequently, Brauer de Marburg developed a positive-pressure device that surrounded only the patient's head, and simplified the operation.

Samuel Meltzer and John Auer, in 1909, introduced the intratracheal positive ventilation

technique, thus eliminating the need for the negative-pressure chamber.[76] Important stages in the development of anesthesia included the following[77]:

- 1869: First endotracheal anesthesia using a tracheotomy cannula by Friedrich Trendelenburg.
- 1880: First orotracheal intubation anesthesia by William Macewen.
- 1894: Positive-pressure ventilation following morphine intoxication by George Fell and Joseph O'Dwyer.

Intraoperative adjustments for thoracic surgery were also developed. One example was patient positioning to mitigate infected secretions from spilling into the noninfected lung. The prone position was adopted as an alternative drainage mechanism to the lateral decubitus position (**Fig. 5**).[78] Other methods included intrabronchial suctioning and bronchial blockers.

Historically, the role of TB drainage has not been well discussed. Hippocrates performed open drainage for empyema.[79] However, in the pre-antibiotic era, it was recommended, especially by Alexander, not to drain TB empyema for fear of opening lateral chest cavities, or contaminating the TB empyema.[72] This unsupported claim continued for many years.

Eloesser[79] advocated open chest drainage for empyema following an open thoracotomy infectious or contaminated space issue (**Fig. 6**). Monaldi[80] advocated open drainage or cavernostomy for other complex situations. One example was a 2-stage procedure for a lateral infected TB cavity.

Restoring negative intrathoracic pressure postoperatively was a major advance. Playfair, in 1873, and Bulau, in 1875, pioneered the water seal drainage system.[81,82] Additional historic TB surgical procedures are noted in **Box 7**.

The growth of competent thoracic surgeons with the skill sets and dedication to the craft was basically a self-learning process, with interested surgeons slowly seeking experienced thoracic surgeons and centers both at home or abroad to

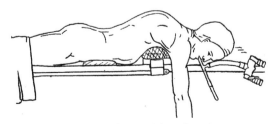

Fig. 5. Prone operative position for thoracotomy. (*From* Parry Brown AI. Posture in thoracic surgery. Thorax 1948;3:164; with permission.)

observe and learn the new techniques and approaches. The learning curve was very steep, given the high early mortality and morbidity rates in the early years. Naef[63] pointed out that the early operations were performed by nonsurgical physicians, yet emerging experienced thoracic surgeons gradually took over. In addition, many of the operations were performed at the sanatoriums, given the fear of performing operations in their own hospital.

The development and reporting of thoracic surgical procedures were difficult to evaluate. The chronology was available, but the caseloads, degree of complexity, timing of the surgery, and selection of a particular procedure were not well recorded or evaluated. There existed an atmosphere of individual preferences, and a paucity of consensus. There was a high learning curve, yet the overall results improved with time.

The early major complications included bronchopleural fistula, sepsis, pulmonary lung dysfunction, and recurrent disease secondary to incomplete lung resection.

Medical Treatment

The major therapeutic modality in the early to middle twentieth century continued to be the sanatorium and surgical treatment. Thereafter, with the development of antibiotics, between 1944 and the early 1950s, surgery declined, as well as the sanatoriums.[83,84]

As noted, most previous medical efforts were not effective. One exception was with bovine tuberculosis that was passed to humans through

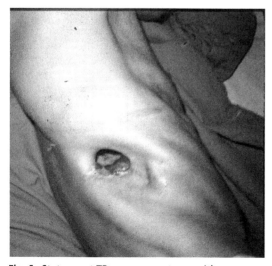

Fig. 6. Status post TB pneumonectomy with empyema and BPF requiring Eloesser flap open drainage. BPF, bronchopleural fistula. (*Courtesy of* A. Thomas Pezzella, MD, Boca Raton, FL.)

infected milk. Pasteurization, started in 1906, eliminated that as a cause of infection, especially in children.[85]

Adequate treatment of TB required a reliable correct diagnosis, as noted with a positive skin test (PPD), positive sputum acid-fast stain (Ziehl-Neelsen) test (number of red snappers per HPF), or the auramine fluorescein stain, and a positive Lowenstein-Jenson medium culture.[51] Other current diagnostic tests included IGRAS-Quanti FERON TB Gold test, and T-Spot TB test.[86]

Following the principles of Louis Pasteur, in 1880, with attenuating the virulence of a living microbe, a vaccine produced with *Mycobacteria bovis* was developed in 1908 by Albert Calmette and Camilo Guerin.[87] They grew the Koch bacillus in several media to decrease its virulence and to increase immunity. The Bacille Calmette Guerin (BCG) vaccine was first used in humans in 1921, and became widely used primarily for children.[87] Currently, there remains no universal totally effective vaccine for TB.

Casadevall,[88] in 2017, discussed the role of vaccines in cell-mediated responses to TB. He postulated that latent TB is more effective in protection and inhibition of the growth of *M tuberculosis* in vitro than active TB. This implies that newer vaccines that promote latency may be more beneficial in infection control.

The timeline for the antibiotic development for TB started in 1935 when Gerhard Domagk published a report on the use of "Prontosil," an organic compound containing sulfur (sulfanilamide), yet it was deemed too toxic for humans. In 1944, a major advance occurred with the discovery of streptomycin (*Streptomyces griseous*) by Schatz, Bugie, and Waksman. It was limited by the early development of resistance. In 1945, para-aminosalicylic acid (PAS) was discovered. When combined with streptomycin, it decreased drug resistance. Following streptomycin, isoniazid (1952), pyrazinamide (1954), ethambutol (1962), and rifampin (rifampicin) (1963) were introduced.[83,84,89–91]

Treatment strategies beyond the drugs depended on prevention, education, social aspects, and compliance, along with access to care, availability, and surveillance. Developed by Karel Styblo with the International Union Against Tuberculosis and Lung Disease in the 1970s, the directly observed treatment, short-course (DOTS) strategy was recommended by the World Health Organization (WHO). In 1995, the WHO adopted the DOTS that focused on cure rates, and limiting the spread of drug resistance. Subsequent trials found significant differences in cure rates or treatment completion between DOTS and self-administered treatment. The WHO continues to use DOTS as an important strategy for TB drug care.[92]

Adjuvant Surgery

Starting in 1944, the need for thoracic TB surgery gradually decreased.[83,84,93–98] However, the recent development of TB-resistant strains, starting in 1980, has created a current need for adjuvant surgery in the complex cases that have increased globally to more than 500,000 new cases per year.

At present, thoracic surgeons in developed countries have had limited or no experience with TB surgery. This is especially true in the United States and Western Europe. The increase of resistant strains, medical failures, the residual sequelae of the disease process, and migration of suspected TB patients from LMICs or EEs, have all created a need for surgical participation that includes surgery in selected cases.

There has been a steady increase in thoracic surgery for patients with TB. The indications, both absolute and relative, have been articulated, as well as the specific surgical approaches and techniques.[93–95] Perioperative aspects, including preoperative selection and preparation, complications, and follow-up results will be further presented and discussed in subsequent articles.

WHO has listed the current operative procedures that are available (**Box 9**).[96] The development of a team approach is now recommended. The team should include thoracic surgeon, infectious disease, pulmonary, and radiology. There remains a global dichotomy in that the developed countries have the technology and resources but less experience, whereas the LMICs and EEs have less modern conveniences but more clinical experience.

Global cooperation between both sectors would be well received and productive, as noted in the recommendations of the WHO Task Force on the role of surgery in MDR-TB.[97]

SUMMARY

Suffice it to say, the treatment and control of TB remains a formable challenge. TB is caused by an infectious bacterium that continues to develop resistant strains. Environmental and social factors, as noted in history, have also played a major role in its persistence, especially in LMICs and EEs. The ongoing global medical solutions alone have not cured or prevented TB. Already there has been a progress movement for the development of TB medical teams composed of

---

> **Box 9**
> **Current modified TB surgical procedures**
>
> - Lung resections of different sizes:
>   - Wedge resection
>   - Segmentectomy
>   - Lobectomy
> - Pneumonectomy or pleuropneumonectomy
> - Extrapleural thoracoplasty (ping pong balls; inflatable silastic pouch)
> - Extrapleural pneumolysis (plombage)
> - Modified thoracoplasty[96]
> - Thoracomyoplasty
> - Pleurectomy and decortication of the lung
> - Operations on the tracheo-bronchial tree:
>   - Occlusion
>   - Resection
>   - Bronchoplasty
>   - Reamputation of the residual stump; open or closed
> - Closed thoracentesis
> - Open window thoracostomy (Eloesser flap)[79]
> - Closed thoracostomy
> - Muscle flaps[99]
> - Mini thoracoplasty[100]

---

pulmonary, infectious disease, and thoracic surgery doctors, as well as public heart physicians. The major challenges include multiple resistant TB, compliance with medical treatment, and the role of surgery to be more involved with medical treatment failures before the exhaustion of medical treatment choices. In addition, TB sequelae and advanced TB resistance will require earlier surgical involvement, as well as being involved earlier with phthisiology team approaches. This will require cooperation of public health, thoracic surgery, infectious disease, and pulmonary medical specialties.

REFERENCES

1. Kipling R. Available at: http://www.kiplingsociety.co.uk/poems_serving.htm. Accessed May 19, 2018.
2. TB. Available at: www.who.int/en/news-room/factsheets/detail/tuberculosis. Accessed May 19, 2018.
3. Bayer R, Castro KG. Tuberculosis elimination in the United States—the need for renewed action. N Engl J Med 2017;377:1109–11.

4. History of tuberculosis. Available at: https://en.wikipedia.org/wiki/History_of_tuberculosis. Accessed February 19, 2018.

5. Daniel TM. The history of tuberculosis. Respir Med 2006;100:1862–70.

6. Frith J. History of tuberculosis. Part 1- phthisis, consumption and the white plague. J Mil Veterans Health 2014;22:30–5.

7. Frith J. History of tuberculosis. Part 2- the sanatoria and the discoveries of the Tubercle Bacillus. J Mil Veterans Health 2014;22:36–41.

8. Barberis I, Bragazzi NL, Martini LG. The history of tuberculosis: from the first historical records to the isolation of Koch's bacillus. J Prev Med Hyg 2017;58:E9–12.

9. First unit: tuberculosis through the history. Available at: https://www.scribd.com/document/7556133/History-of-Tuberculosis. Accessed May 19, 2018.

10. Ringer PH. The evolution of the treatment of pulmonary tuberculosis. Chest 1938;4:8–13.

11. Shampo MA, Rosenow EC. A history of tuberculosis on stamps. Chest 2009;136:578–82.

12. Davies, PDO. A little history of tuberculosis. Available at: http://www.evolve360.co.uk/Data/10/Docs/19/19Davies.pdf. Accessed October 7, 2018.

13. Lauer SA. The social impact of the misconceptions surrounding tuberculosis. Iowa Historical Review 2017;7:55–78.

14. McKeown RE. The epidemiologic transition: changing patterns of mortality and population dynamics. Am J Lifestyle Med 2009;3(1 Suppl):19S–26S.

15. Omran AR. The epidemiologic transition. A theory of the epidemiology of population change. Milbank Mem Fund Q 1971;49:509–38.

16. Gersh BJ, Sliwa K, Mayosi BM, et al. The epidemic of cardiovascular disease in the developing world: global implications. Eur Heart J 2010;31:642–8.

17. Economic evolution, diversity of societies and stages of economic development: A critique of theories applied to hunters and gatherers and their successors. Available at: https://www.researchgate.net/publication/299338207_Economic_evolution_diversity_of_societies_and_stages_of_economic_development_A_critique_of_theories_applied_to_hunters_and_gatherers_and_their_successors. Accessed October 7, 2018.

18. Tuberculosis fact sheet. Available at: http://www.who.int/mediacentre/factsheets/fs104/en/. Accessed May 19, 2018.

19. Global tuberculosis report 2017. Available at: http://www.who.int/tb/publications/global_report/gtbr2017_main_text.pdf. Accessed May 19, 2018.

20. GBD 2015 mortality and cause of death collaborators. Global, regional, and national life expectancy, all-cause mortality, and cause-specific mortality for 249 causes of death, 1980-2015: a systematic analysis for the Global Burdon of Disease Study 2015. Lancet 2016; 388:1459–544.

21. GBD 2016 DALYs, HALE Collaborators. Global, regional, and national disability-adjusted life-years (DALYs) for 333 diseases and injuries and healthy life expectancy (HALE) for 195 countries and territories, 1990–2016: a systematic analysis for the global burden of disease study 2016. Lancet 2017;390:1260–344.

22. Smith I. *Mycobacterium tuberculosis* pathogenesis and molecular determinants of virulence. Clin Microbiol Rev 2003;16:463–96.

23. Tuberculosis. Available at: https://en.wikipedia.org/wiki/Tuberculosis. Accessed May 19, 2018.

24. Roy CJ, Milton DK. Airborne transmission of communicable infection—the elusive pathway. N Engl J Med 2004;350:1710–2.

25. Datta M, Via LE, Chen W, et al. Mathematical model of oxygen transport in tuberculosis. Ann Biomed Eng 2016;44:863–72.

26. Rothschild BM, Martin LD, Lev G, et al. *Mycobacterium tuberculosis* complex DNA from an extinct bison dated 17,000 years before the present. Clin Infect Dis 2001;33:305–11.

27. Hershkovitz I, Donoghue HD, Minnikin DE, et al. Detection and molecular characterization of 9000-year-old *Mycobacterium tuberculosis* from a neolithic settlement in the Eastern Mediterranean. PLoS One 2008;3:e3426.

28. Nicklisch N, Maixner F, Ganslmeier R, et al. Rib lesions in skeletons from early neolithic sites in Central Germany: on the trail of tuberculosis at the onset of agriculture. Am J Phys Anthropol 2012; 149:391–404.

29. Bos KI, Harkins KM, Krause J. Pre-Columbian mycobacterial genomes reveal seals as a source of New World human tuberculosis. Nature 2014; 51:494–7.

30. Gagneux S. Host-pathogen coevolution in human tuberculosis. Philos Trans R Soc Lond B Biol Sci 2012;367:850–9.

31. Gutierrez MC, Brisse S, Brosch R, et al. Ancient origin and gene mosaicism of the progenitor of *Mycobacterium tuberculosis*. PLoS Pathog 2005; 1:0055–61.

32. Wirth T, Hildebrand F, Allix-Beguec C, et al. Origin, spread and demography of the *Mycobacterium tuberculosis* complex. PLoS Pathog 2008;4: el000160.

33. Woolhouse MEJ, Webster JP, Domingo E, et al. Biological and biomedical implications of the co-evolution of pathogens and their host. Nat Genet 2002;32:569–77.

34. Muller R, Roberts CA, Brown TA. Genotyping of ancient *Mycobacterium tuberculosis* strains reveals historic genetic diversity. Proc Biol Sci 2014;281:20133236.

35. Namouchi A, Didelot X, Shock U, et al. After the bottle-neck: genome-wide diversification of the *Mycobacterium* complex by mutation, recombination, and natural selection. Genome Res 2012;22:721–34.

36. CDC-TB chronicle. Available at: https://www.cdc.gov/tb/worldtbday/history.htm. Accessed May 19, 2018.

37. Timeline of tuberculosis. Available at: https://en.wikipedia.org/wiki/Timeline_of_tuberculosis. Accessed May 19, 2018.

38. Daniel VS, Daniel TM. Old Testament biblical reference to tuberculosis. Clin Infect Dis 1999;29:1557–8.

39. Hippocrates & Galen - the four humors. Available at: http://paei.wikidot.com/hippocrates-galen-the-four-humors. Accessed May 19, 2018.

40. Laios K, Androutsos G, Moschos MM. Aretaeus of Cappadocia and pulmonary tuberculosis. Balkan Med J 2017;34:480. Available at: https://www.ncbi.nlm.nih.gov/pmc/articles/PMC5635640/. Accessed May 19, 2018.

41. Galen. Available at: https://en.wikipedia.org/wiki/Galen#Influence_on_medicine_in_the_Islamic_world. Accessed October 7, 2018.

42. Tuberculosis and the vampire myth. Available at: http://www.aeras.org/blog/tuberculosis-and-the-vampire-myth#.Wr0lgy7w. Accessed May 18, 2018.

43. Paracelsus. Available at: https://en.wikipedia.org/wiki/Paracelsus. Accessed May 18, 2018.

44. Tuberculosis in Europe and North America, 1800–1922. Available at: http://ocp.hul.harvard.edu/contagion/tuberculosis.html. Accessed May 19, 2018.

45. TB sheets. Available at: https://www.azlyrics.com/lyrics/vanmorrison/tbsheets.html. Accessed May 19, 2018.

46. CDC -History of world TB day. TB chronicles. Available at: https://www.cdc.gov/tb/worldtbday/history.htm. Accessed May 18, 2018.

47. Koch's postulates. Available at: https://www.google.com/search?q=koch%27s+postulates&rlz=1C1TSNP_enUS484US582&source=lnms&tbm=isch&sa=X&ved=0ahUKEwjL67KqldHaAhUKo4MKHdr7DDkQ_AUICigB&biw=1366&bih=662#imgrc=3EodcznKRhy_M. Accessed May 19, 2018.

48. German scientist discovers X-rays, 1895. Available at: https://www.nde-ed.org/EducationResources/HighSchool/Radiography/discoveryxrays.htm. Accessed May 19, 2018.

49. Mantoux test. Available at: https://en.wikipedia.org/wiki/Mantoux_test. Accessed May 19, 2018.

50. Leopold Auenbrugger. Available at: https://en.wikipedia.org/wiki/Leopold_Auenbrugger. Accessed May 19, 2018.

51. Löwenstein–Jensen medium. Available at: https://en.wikipedia.org/wiki/L%C3%B6wenstein%E2%80%93Jensen_mediumm. Accessed May 19, 2018.

52. Confinement in a facility. Available at: https://www.cdc.gov/tb/programs/laws/menu/confinement.htm. Accessed May 19, 2018.

53. Planning the Nation: the sanatorium movement in Germany. Available at: https://www.tandfonline.com/doi/full/10.1080/13602365.2014.966587?scroll=top&needAccess=true. Accessed May 21, 2018.

54. The Sanatorium Movement in America. Available at: http://scalar.usc.edu/hc/tuberculosis-exhibit/the-sanatorium-movement-in-america. Accessed May 21, 2018.

55. Fitzsimons General Hospital. Available at: https://coloradoencyclopedia.org/article/fitzsimons-general-hospital. Accessed May 19, 2018.

56. Inzirillo F, Tiberi S, Donati M, et al. Surgical treatment of tuberculosis, yesterday and today. SMGrup; 2016. Available at: http://www.smgebooks.com/tuberculosis/chapters/TB-16-10.pdf. Accessed October 6, 2018.

57. The sanatorium files: Part 3 – the sanatorium movement. Available at: http://www.newtbdrugs.org/news/sanatorium-files-part-3-%E2%80%93-sanatorium-movement. Accessed May 22, 2018.

58. The magic mountain. Available at: https://www.enotes.com/topics/magic-mountain. Accessed May 22, 2018.

59. Chaikhouni A. The magnificent century of cardiothoracic surgery. Heart Views 2008;9:86–90.

60. Hurt R. The history of cardiothoracic surgery from early time. London; The Parthenon Publishing Group; 1996. p. 153–82, 203–23.

61. Pezzella AT, Fang W. Surgical aspects of thoracic tuberculosis: a contemporary review- part 1. Curr Probl Surg 2008;45:669–758.

62. Odell JA. History of surgery for pulmonary tuberculosis. Thorac Surg Clin 2012;22:257–69.

63. Naef AP. The 1900 tuberculosis epidemic—starting point of modern thoracic surgery. Ann Thorac Surg 1993;55:1375–8.

64. Mehran RJ, Deslauriers J. Tuberculosis and atypical mycobacterial diseases. In: Patterson GA, Cooper JD, Deslauriers J, et al, editors. Pearson's thoracic & esophageal surgery. 3rd edition. Philadelphia: Churchill Livingstone/Elsevier; 2008. p. 499–505.

65. Sakula A. Carlo Forlanini, inventor of artificial pneumothorax for treatment of pulmonary tuberculosis. Thorax 1983;38:326–32.

66. Rakovich G. Artificial pneumothorax: tapping into a small bit of history. CMAJ 2010;182:179.

67. Long ER. Artificial pneumothorax in tuberculosis. Am J Nurs 1919;19:265–8.

68. Loddenkemper R, Mathur PN, Lee P, et al. History and clinical use of thoroscopy/pleuroscopy in respiratory medicine. Breath 2011;8:145–55.

69. Steele JD. The surgical treatment of pulmonary tuberculosis. Ann Thorac Surg 1968;6:485–502.

70. Alexander J. The surgery of pulmonary tuberculosis. Philadelphia: Lea and Febiger; 1925.

71. Alexander J. The collapse therapy of pulmonary tuberculosis. Springfield (IL): Charles C. Thomas; 1937.

72. Langston HT. Thoracoplasty: the how and the why. Ann Thorac Surg 1991;52:1351–3.

73. Weissberg D, Weissberg D. Late complications of collapse therapy. Chest 2001;120:847–51.

74. Dung LT, Luan TMB, Pezzella AT. Thoracic plombage procedure for tuberculosis/aspergillosis abscess cavity. Africa. Ann Thorac Cardiovasc Surg 2013;8:52–8.

75. Walcott-Sapp S, Sukumar M. The history of pulmonary lobectomy: two phases of innovation. CTSNet. Available at: https://www.ctsnet.org/article/history-pulmonary-lobectomy-two-phases-innovation. Accessed May 19, 2018.

76. Meltzer A. Dr. Samuel James Meltzer and intratracheal anesthesia. J Clin Anesth 1990;2:54–8.

77. The history of endotracheal anesthesia, with special regard to the development of the endotracheal tube. Available at: https://www.ncbi.nlm.nih.gov/pubmed/3535566. Accessed May 19, 2018.

78. Parry Brown AI. Posture in thoracic surgery. Thorax 1948;3:161–5.

79. Eloesser L. Of an operation for tuberculous empyema. Ann Thorac Surg 1969;8:355–7.

80. Monaldi VA. Propos du procede d'aspiration intra-cavitair des caverns. Rev Tuberc 1939;5: 848–56.

81. Walcott-Sapp S, Sukumar M. A history of thoracic drainage: from ancient Greeks to wound sucking drummers to digital monitoring. Available at: http://www.ctsnet.org/article/history-thoracic-drainage-ancient-greeks-wound-sucking-drummers-digital-monitoring. Accessed May 21, 2018.

82. Meyer JA. Gotthard Bulau and closed water-seal drainage for empyema—875-1891. Ann Thorac Surg 1989;48:597–9.

83. Murray JF. A century of tuberculosis. Am J Respir Crit Care Med 2004;169:1181–6.

84. Murray JF. Treatment of tuberculosis. A historical perspective. Ann Am Thorac Soc 2015;12: 1749–59.

85. Pasteurization. Available at: https://en.wikipedia.org/wiki/Pasteurization#History. Accessed May 19, 2018.

86. TB elimination. Available at: https://www.cdc.gov/tb/publications/factsheets/testing/IGRA.pdf. Accessed October 7, 2018.

87. BCG vaccine. Available at: https://en.wikipedia.org/wiki/BCG_vaccine. Accessed May 19, 2018.

88. Casadevall A. Antibodies to *Mycobacterium tuberculosis*. N Engl J Med 2017;376:283–5.

89. Callgaro GL, Moodley L, Symons G, et al. The medical and surgical treatment of drug-resistant tuberculosis. J Thorac Dis 2014;6(3):189–95.

90. TB facts: history of TB drugs – PAS, streptomycin, Waksman. Available at: https://www.tbfacts.org/history-of-tb-drugs/. Accessed May 19, 2018.

91. Tuberculosis management. Available at: https://en.wikipedia.org/wiki/Tuberculosis_managementhttps://en.wikipedia.org/wiki/Tuberculosis_management. Accessed May 19m, 2018.

92. Directly observed treatment, short-course. Available at: https://en.wikipedia.org/wiki/Directly_observed_treatment,_short-course. Accessed May 19, 2018.

93. Tuberculosis history. Available at: https://www.nationaljewish.org/conditions/tuberculosis-tb/history. Accessed May 19, 2018.

94. Kempker RR, Vashakidze S, Solomonia N, et al. Grand round calling the surgeon: the role of surgery in the treatment of drug-resistant tuberculosis. Lancet Infect Dis 2012;12:157–66.

95. Subotic D, Yablonskiy P, Sulis G, et al. Surgery and pleuro-pulmonary tuberculosis: a scientific literature review. J Thorac Dis 2016;8:E474–85.

96. WHO- The role of surgery in the treatment of pulmonary TB and multidrug- and extensively drug resistant TB. Available at: http://www.euro.who.int/__data/assets/pdf_file/0005/259691/The-role-of-surgery-in-the-treatment-of-pulmonary-TB-and-multidrug-and-extensively-drug-resistant-TB.pdf. Accessed May 21, 2018.

97. Chakaya J. Long term complications after completion of pulmonary tuberculosis treatment: a quest for a public health approach. J Clin Tuberc Other Mycobact Dis 2016;3:10–2.

98. Pomerantz BJ, Cleveland JC, Pomerantz M. The schede and modern thoracoplasty. Oper Tech Thorac Cardiovasc Surg 2000;5:128–34.

99. Harris SU, Nahai F. Intrathoracic muscle transposition. Chest Surg Clin N Am 1996;6:501–18.

100. Krasnov D, Krasnov V, Skvortsov D, et al. Thoracoplasty for tuberculosis in the twenty-first century. Thorac Surg Clin 2017;27:99–111.

The Global Fight Against Tuberculosis

Charles L. Daley, MD

KEYWORDS

- Mycobacterium tuberculosis • Epidemiology • Global control • Drug resistant

KEY POINTS

- An estimated 1.7 billion (23%) of the world's population is infected with *Mycobacterium tuberculosis* leading to more than 10 million new tuberculosis (TB) cases each year.
- TB is one of the top 10 causes of death globally and is the leading cause of death from a single infectious disease agent.
- In 2016, there were 600,000 new cases of TB resistant to rifampicin, of which 490,000 had multidrug resistant TB.
- The World Health Organization's ambitious End TB Strategy aims to achieve a 95% reduction in TB deaths and 90% reduction in TB incidence rates by 2035.
- The End TB Strategy is anchored by 3 pillars: (1) integrated, patient-centered care and prevention; (2) bold policies and supportive systems; and (3) intensified research and innovation.

INTRODUCTION

Tuberculosis (TB) continues to ravage the world leading to tremendous morbidity and mortality. An estimated 1.7 billion (23%) of the world's population is infected with *Mycobacterium tuberculosis* leading to more than 10 million new cases each year.[1] TB is one of the top 10 causes of death globally and is the leading cause of death from a single infectious disease agent, resulting in 1.7 million deaths annually, including 0.4 million among people living with human immunodeficiency virus infection (HIV).[2] Sadly, most of these deaths could be averted with earlier diagnosis and treatment. This article reviews the global epidemiology of TB, including drug-resistant disease as well as the actions being taken at a global level to curtail and eventually eliminate the disease.

GLOBAL EPIDEMIOLOGY OF TUBERCULOSIS

In 2016, there were an estimated 10.4 million new (or incident) cases of TB worldwide, of which approximately 10% were in HIV-infected individuals.[2] Ninety percent of the cases were in adults and 65% in men. The burden of disease varies significantly by World Health Organization (WHO) Region, with approximately 45% of the new cases in the WHO South-East Asian Region followed by the African Region (25%), Eastern Mediterranean Region (7%), European Region (3%), and Region of the Americas (3%) (**Fig. 1**). Approximately half of these estimated cases are from 5 countries, including India, Indonesia, China, Philippines, and Pakistan. The WHO has focused its efforts on countries with a high burden of disease including countries with a high burden of TB, multidrug resistant TB (MDR-TB), and HIV-TB: 14 countries are in each list (**Fig. 2**).

Disclosure: Otsuka, Member, Data Monitoring Committee for delamanid.
Division of Mycobacterial and Respiratory Infections, National Jewish Health, 1400 Jackson Street, Denver, CO 80206, USA
E-mail address: daleyc@njhealth.org

Thorac Surg Clin 29 (2019) 19–25
https://doi.org/10.1016/j.thorsurg.2018.09.010

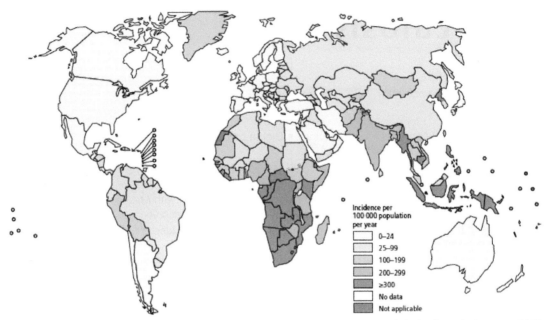

Fig. 1. Estimated TB incidence rates, 2016. (*From* World Health Organization. Global tuberculosis report 2017. Geneva (Switzerland): World Health Organization; 2017; with permission.)

Among the estimated new TB cases, only 6.3 million (61%) were reported to TB programs in 2016.[2] Ten countries accounted for 76% of this gap between estimated and notified cases; the top 3 were India (25%), Indonesia (16%), and Nigeria (8%). The TB incidence has been declining globally at about 1.4% per year between 2000 and 2016 with a 1.9% decline in 2015 to 2016. At this rate of decline it would take more than a century to achieve elimination of TB.

TB continues to result in unnecessary deaths. There were an estimated 1.3 million deaths among HIV-negative people in 2016, which made TB the ninth leading cause of death and for the past 5 years, the leading cause of death from a single infectious disease agent.[2,3] However, like TB incidence, there are large variations in the TB mortality rate ranging from 1 TB death per 100,000 population in many high-income countries to 40 or more deaths per 100,000 population in the WHO African Region and in 5 high burden countries.[2] Of the 1.3 million total deaths, WHO estimated that 0.4 million HIV-infected people died of TB, making it the leading cause of death among those living with HIV. Fortunately, the number of deaths has been falling since 2000, with a 3% per year decline between 2015 and 2016. Treatment of TB can prevent most of these deaths. WHO estimates that TB treatment averted 44 million deaths among HIV-negative people between 2000 and 2016 and that TB treatment plus antiretroviral therapy averted 8.5 million deaths among HIV-positive people.[2]

Drug-resistant TB continues to threaten global TB control. In 2016, there were 600,000 new cases of TB resistant to rifampicin (RR-TB), of which 490,000 had MDR-TB defined as resistance to at least isoniazid and rifampicin.[2] Approximately half of these cases occurred in India (25%), China (12%), and the Russian Federation (10%). Globally, an estimated 4.1% of new cases and 19% of previously treated cases had MDR-TB.[2] Approximately 6% of MDR-TB patients had additional resistance to the fluoroquinolones and at least one second-line injectable, referred to as extensively resistant TB (XDR-TB): 123 countries had reported at least 1 case of XDR-TB.[2] MDR and XDR-TB are difficult to treat and associated with poor treatment outcomes, including high mortality rates, in most programmatic settings: there were an estimated 240,000 deaths from MDR/RR-TB in 2016 similar to that reported in 2015.

GLOBAL STRATEGY TO END TUBERCULOSIS

The WHO declared TB as a global emergency in 1993 after a period of prolonged neglect.[4] TB-related indicators were established by the United Nations (UN) 2000 to 2015 Millennium Development Goals (MDGs) with the aim of reversing the TB incidence. The Stop TB Partnership developed 2 additional targets including reducing TB prevalence and mortality by 50% by 2015 compared

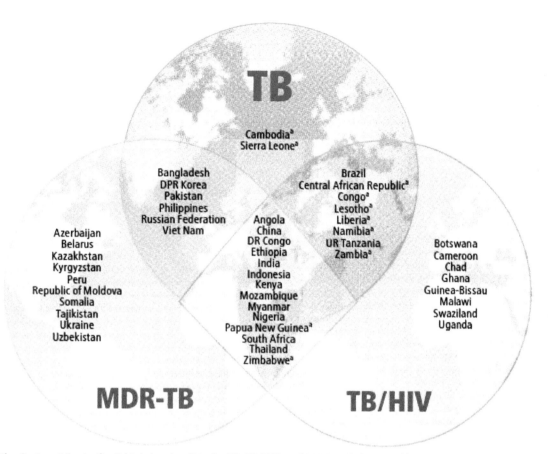

Fig. 2. Countries in the 3 high burden lists for TB, TB/HIV, and MDR-TB being used by WHO during the period 2016 to 2020, and their areas of overlap. [a] Countries that are included in the list of 30 high burden TB countries on the basis of severity of their TB burden (ie, TB incidence per 100,000 population), as opposed to the top 20, which are included based on their absolute number of incident cases per year. (*From* World Health Organization. Global tuberculosis report 2017. Geneva (Switzerland): World Health Organization; 2017; with permission.)

with 1990. In order to achieve the MDGs, the WHO developed and implemented a series of TB control strategies, including the DOTS Strategy (2000–2005) and Stop TB Strategy (2006–15). Based on the recent UN 2016 to 2030 Sustainable Development Goals, the WHO has embarked on the End TB Strategy that covers the period 2016 to 2035.[4]

The End TB Strategy was formulated for post-2015 global TB control. The Vision of the strategy is a world free of TB with zero deaths, disease, and suffering from TB.[4] The goal is to end the global TB epidemic. In order to measure progress in achievement of this goal, the WHO developed a set of milestones and targets for 2025 and 2035, respectively. The milestones are

1. 75% reduction in TB deaths (compared with 2015),
2. 50% reduction in TB incidence rate, and
3. No affected families facing catastrophic costs due to TB.

The 2035 targets are

1. 95% reduction in TB deaths,
2. 90% reduction in TB incidence rates (<10 cases per 100,000), and
3. No affected families facing catastrophic costs due to TB.

The End TB Strategy is anchored by 3 pillars:

1. Integrated, patient-centered care and prevention,
2. Bold policies and supportive systems, and
3. Intensified research and innovation.[4]

Key actions under Pillar 1 include early diagnosis of TB including the availability of universal drug-susceptibility testing and systematic screening of contacts and high-risk groups. In addition, treatment of all people with TB including drug-resistant TB as well as patient support should be provided. Collaboration between TB and HIV activities is recommended along with

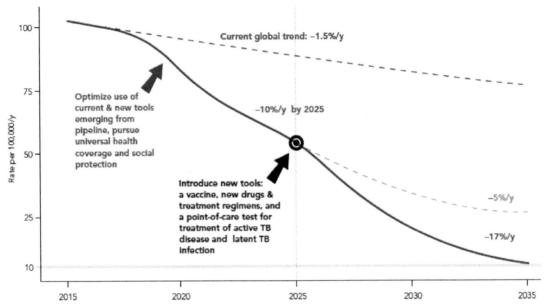

Fig. 3. Projected acceleration in the decline of global TB incidence rates to target levels. (*From* World Health Organization. The end TB strategy. Geneva (Switzerland): World Health Organization; 2014; with permission.)

management of comorbidities, such as diabetes mellitus, and finally, preventive treatment of persons at high risk of progressing to TB disease. Pillar 2 calls for bold policies and supportive systems that require political commitment with adequate resources for TB care and prevention as well as community engagement. Critical to achieving the components of Pillar 2 is the provision of universal health coverage and adequate regulatory frameworks for case notification, vital registration, as well as quality and rational use of medicines and infection control. Pillar 3 calls for intensified research and innovation. Two components of this pillar include discovery, development, and rapid uptake of new tools, interventions, and strategies as well as research to optimize implementation and impact of these tools.[4]

Achieving the milestones and targets of the End TB Strategy will not be easy. To achieve the 2020 and 2025 milestones the global rate of decline in TB incidence must accelerate from 1.5% per year to 4% to 5% per year by 2020 and to 10% per year by 2025 (**Fig. 3**).[3] The proportion of people who die from TB must be reduced from 17% in 2015 to 10% by 2020 and 6.5% in 2025.[3] In order to achieve these ambitious targets, we will need to optimize the use of current tools and introduce new tools such as vaccines, new drugs, and regimens and treat both active and latent TB infection (LTBI). The latter intervention, treatment of LTBI, will be a critical but challenging component of the strategy to implement at a global level.[5]

CURRENT APPROACH TO GLOBAL TUBERCULOSIS CONTROL

The WHO has published numerous policy statements and guidelines with the aim of improving the diagnosis, treatment, and care of patients with TB. The WHO published a "Compendium" that consolidates all current WHO TB policy recommendations into a single source.[6] The "Compendium" includes 33 standards that provide a framework to achieve the targets of the End TB Strategy. By following these standards, we should be able to move closer to achieving the goals of the End TB Strategy.

Early Detection and Diagnosis of Tuberculosis

For persons with signs and symptoms consistent with TB, performing prompt clinical evaluation is essential to ensure early and rapid diagnosis.[7] To diagnose TB efficiently and accurately, a functional, tiered network of quality-assured, integrated laboratories with appropriate biosafety measures in place is required.[4,8,9] Despite significant advances in molecular diagnostics, TB is still usually diagnosed with acid-fast bacillus smear and cultures.[10] The WHO recommends that all patients suspected of having TB, who can produce sputum, have at least 1 sputum specimen submitted for Xpert MTB/RIF Ultra assay.[8] This includes children who are able to produce sputum. A second specimen may be submitted in those whose test is initially negative by Xpert but whose signs and symptoms persist. Xpert MTB/RIF Ultra assay can provide a rapid diagnosis of TB as well as detect the presence of rifampicin resistance. Drug susceptibility testing using rapid molecular tests should be used in all patients. If RR-TB is detected, rapid molecular tests should be performed to detect resistance to isoniazid, fluoroquinolones, and second-line injectables.[11,12] Culture-based susceptibility testing is still useful against drugs for which molecular tests are not yet available. The End TB Strategy calls for universal drug susceptibility testing; however, in 2016, rifampicin resistance was detected in only 33% of newly diagnosed cases and 60% of those previously treated.[4] This is unacceptably low coverage and likely explains why most of the estimated 350,000 cases of drug-resistant TB among notified cases were undetected.

Treatment of Tuberculosis

Drug-susceptible TB is treated with a 6-month regimen that includes isoniazid, rifampicin, ethambutol, and pyrazinamide for the first 2 months followed by isoniazid and rifampicin in the subsequent 4 months.[13,14] Treatment outcomes reported to the WHO have demonstrated success rates of 80% to 86% since 2000.[3] Corticosteroids are recommended by the WHO as adjunctive therapy in patients with TB meningitis or pericarditis. The American Thoracic Society also recommends corticosteroids for TB meningitis but not for pericarditis.[13] Unfortunately, attempts to shorten therapy to 4 months have been unsuccessful.[15–18]

RR-TB and MDR-TB are treated with a regimen that includes at least 5 likely active drugs including a fluoroquinolone and second-line injectable drug, when possible.[19] The intensive phase is administered for 8 months and the total duration of therapy is at least 20 months. Treatment outcomes are much worse than for drug-susceptible disease: treatment success is 54% for MDR-TB and 30% for XDR-TB.[2] New drugs and treatment regimens have been introduced that have been associated with improved treatment outcomes and improved tolerance compared with traditional MDR-TB regimens.[19–22] Whenever possible, these new drugs should be added to MDR-TB regimens in order to include at least 5 active drugs.

Since 2016, the WHO has recommended shorter regimens (9–12 months), which include 7 drugs.[19,23] An observational study from Bangladesh reported a treatment success rate of 88% using this regimen.[24] Subsequent studies from 9 African countries reported similarly high success rates of 82%.[25]

In some patients, antimicrobial therapy is insufficient for durable cure. In selected patients with focal disease, surgical resection should be considered.[19]

Diagnosis and Treatment of Latent Tuberculosis Infection

Achieving TB elimination will not be possible without an effective new vaccine and/or treatment of LTBI. Modeling studies have demonstrated that the most effective way to decrease the incidence of TB is to diagnosis and treat both TB and LTBI.[5] The tuberculin skin test (TST) has been the standard test for diagnosing LTBI; however, newer interferon gamma release assays (IGRAs) are now available, including QuantiFERON and T-SPOT.TB.[10] For diagnosis of LTBI, the WHO recommends that either a TST or an interferon gamma release assay be used. However, in individuals vaccinated with BCG, the IGRAs are clearly superior to the TST.[10] In patients with HIV infection or children younger than 5 years, a positive TST or IGRA is not required to initiate preventive therapy given the high risk of progression to active TB.

Treatment regimens for LTBI include isoniazid for 6 to 9 months, rifampicin for 4 months, isoniazid and rifampicin for 3 to 4 months, or isoniazid and rifapentine once weekly for 3 months.[26] The latter regimen provides a shorter course that has been demonstrated to be of similar efficacy to 9 months of isoniazid.[27] The greatest challenge to treatment of LTBI is the prolonged treatment duration. The newer shorter course regimens such as rifampicin for 4 months[28] or isoniazid and rifapentine for 3 months[27] are associated with a significantly higher completion rate and similar efficacy to longer isoniazid regimens. The 3-month regimen of isoniazid and rifapentine regimen administered once weekly has been demonstrated to be effective in HIV-infected individuals[29] as well as children.[30]

CLOSING THE GAPS

As is evident from the WHO reports, there are several gaps in TB control that need to be closed in order to reach the end of TB. Globally, among the estimated 10.1 million new TB cases each year, only 61% were notified to public health programs. Almost 76% of the total global gap between estimated and notified TB cases is accounted for by 10 countries, the top 3 of which are India (25%), Indonesia (16%), and Nigeria (8%). Underreporting and underdiagnosis account for much of this gap.[3] Underreporting is likely a significant contributor in countries where many patients are seen in the private sector. For example, in India and Indonesia, up to half of detected cases might go unreported.[2] Underdiagnosis occurs, either because of failure to detect TB in patients with the disease or because TB patients are not seeking care. Another important gap is that between the estimated incidence and enrollment into treatment. Ten countries accounted for 75% of this gap.[2,3] In 2016, 129,689 people were started on treatment for drug-resistant TB, which was only 22% of the estimated incidence.[3]

India, the country that accounts for the largest number of cases and the largest number of "missing cases," provides a good example of the problems encountered in the "cascade of care" for TB.[2] A systematic review evaluated the TB cascade of care in India and reported that among approximately 2,700,000 prevalent patients with TB, 60% were successfully diagnosed with TB, 53% had started on therapy, 45% of patients with TB completed therapy, and only 39% were disease free after 1 year.[31] The cascade of care in MDR-TB was even worse. Of those diagnosed with MDR-TB, only 14% completed treatment and 11% remained disease free at 1 year. This study found that for patients with smear-negative TB and MDR-TB, increasing detection and diagnosis of new patients by using new TB diagnostic tests may be the most important intervention for improving patient outcomes whereas among new smear positive cases, reducing loss to follow-up and improving adherence may be most effective. In addition, this study highlighted that interventions to improve treatment outcomes will vary across settings and patient populations.

THE WAY FORWARD

In order to accomplish the goals of the End TB Strategy, an infusion of funding and resources is needed. The funding required to address the epidemic in low- and middle-income countries is estimated to be $9.2 billion US dollars.[4] Unfortunately, the current gap is around $2 billion dollars. International donor funding remains critical, accounting for 48% of the funding available for the 25 high TB burden countries (not include BRICS countries) and 56% of funding in low-income countries.

The Stop TB Partnership has issued The Global Plan to End TB, which represents a costed plan for implementation of the first 5 years of the End TB Strategy.[32] The Global Plan introduced 3 people-centered targets called the 90-(90)-90 targets, which are to reach 90% of all people who need TB treatment including 90% of people in key populations and achieve at least 90% treatment success. The plan calls for a "paradigm shift" in the

approach to TB control including 8 fundamental changes:

1. A change in mindset
2. A human-rights and gender-based approach to TB
3. Changed and more inclusive leadership
4. Community- and patient-driven approach
5. Innovative TB programs equipped to end TB
6. Integrated health systems fit for purpose
7. New, innovative, and optimized approach to funding TB care
8. Investment in socioeconomic actions

In order to achieve these targets, a significant increase in resources will be needed. The Global Plan estimates that a total of $56 to 58 billion USD will be needed for implementing TB programs and $9 billion for research and development for new tools. Most of the money would be for operational and health system costs followed by drugs, diagnostics, and management of MDR-TB. Investing in the Plan would save lives, prevent suffering, and ultimately save money.

REFERENCES

1. Houben RM, Dodd PJ. The global burden of latent tuberculosis infection: a re-estimation using mathematical modelling. PLoS Med 2016;13(10): e1002152.
2. World Health Organization. Global tuberculosis control: WHO report 2017. Geneva (Switzerland): 2017.
3. Floyd K, Glaziou P, Zumla A, et al. The global tuberculosis epidemic and progress in care, prevention, and research: an overview in year 3 of the End TB era. Lancet Respir Med 2018;6(4):299–314.
4. WHO. The end TB strategy. Geneva (Switzerland): World Health Organization; 2014.
5. Dye C, Glaziou P, Floyd K, et al. Prospects for tuberculosis elimination. Annu Rev Public Health 2013;34: 271–86.
6. Gilpin C, Korobitsyn A, Migliori GB, et al. The World Health Organization standards for tuberculosis care and management. Eur Respir J 2018;51(3).
7. World Health Organization. Early detection of tuberculosis: an overview of approaches, guidelines and tools. Geneva (Switzerland): World Health Organization; 2018.
8. World Health Organization. Implementing tuberculosis diagnostics: policy framework. Geneva (Switzerland): World Health Organization; 2015.
9. WHO meeting report of a technical expert consultation: non-inferiority analysis of Xpert MTB/RIF ultra compared to Xpert MTB/RIF. Geneva (Switzerland): World Health Organization; 2017.
10. Lewinsohn DM, Leonard MK, LoBue PA, et al. Official American Thoracic Society/Infectious Diseases

Society of America/Centers for Disease Control and Prevention clinical practice guidelines: diagnosis of tuberculosis in adults and children. Clin Infect Dis 2017;64(2):e1–33.

11. World Health Organization. The use of molecular line probe assays for the detection of resistance to isoniazid and rifampicin: policy update. Geneva (Switzerland): World Health Organization; 2016.

12. World Health Organization. The use of molecular line probe assays for the detection of resistance to second line anti-tuberculosis drugs: policy guideance. Geneva (Switzerland): World Health Organization; 2016.

13. Nahid P, Dorman SE, Alipanah N, et al. Official American Thoracic Society/Centers for Disease Control and Prevention/Infectious Diseases Society of America clinical practice guidelines: treatment of drug-susceptible tuberculosis. Clin Infect Dis 2016; 63(7):e147–95.

14. World Health Organization. Treatment of tuberculosis. Guidelines for treatment of drug-susceptible tuberculosis and patient care. Geneva (Switzerland): World Health Organization; 2017.

15. Gillespie SH, Crook AM, McHugh TD, et al. Four-month moxifloxacin-based regimens for drug-sensitive tuberculosis. N Engl J Med 2014;371(17): 1577–87.

16. Merle CS, Fielding K, Sow OB, et al. A four-month gatifloxacin-containing regimen for treating tuberculosis. N Engl J Med 2014;371(17):1588–98.

17. Jindani A, Harrison TS, Nunn AJ, et al. High-dose rifapentine with moxifloxacin for pulmonary tuberculosis. N Engl J Med 2014;371(17):1599–608.

18. Jawahar MS, Banurekha VV, Paramasivan CN, et al. Randomized clinical trial of thrice-weekly 4-month moxifloxacin or gatifloxacin containing regimens in the treatment of new sputum positive pulmonary tuberculosis patients. PLoS One 2013;8(7):e67030.

19. World Health Organization. WHO treatment guidelines for drug-resistant tuberculosis, 2016 update. Geneva (Switzerland): 2016. Report No.: 9789241549639.

20. The use of bedaquiline in the treatment of multidrug-resistant tuberculosis: interim policy guidance. Geneva (Switzerland): World Health Organization; 2013. Report No.: 9789241505482.

21. World Health Organization. The use of delamanid in the treatment of multidrug-resistant tuberculosis: interim policy guidance. Geneva (Switzerland): World Health Organization; 2014.

22. World Health Organization. The use of delamanid in the treatment of multidrug-resistant tuberculosis in children and adolescents: interim policy guidance. Geneva (Switzerland): World Health Organization; 2016. Report No.: 9789241549899.

23. World Health Organization. Position statement on the continued use of the shorter MDR-TB regimen following an expedited review of the STREAM Stage 1 preliminary results. Geneva (Switzerland): 2018.

24. Van Deun A, Maug AK, Salim MA, et al. Short, highly effective, and inexpensive standardized treatment of multidrug-resistant tuberculosis. Am J Respir Crit Care Med 2010;182(5):684–92.

25. Trebucq A, Schwoebel V, Kashongwe Z, et al. Treatment outcome with a short multidrug-resistant tuberculosis regimen in nine African countries. Int J Tuberc Lung Dis 2018;22(1):17–25.

26. World Health Organization. Latent tuberculosis infection: updated and consolidated guidelines for programmatic management. Geneva (Switzerland): World Health Organization; 2018.

27. Sterling TR, Villarino ME, Borisov AS, et al. Three months of rifapentine and isoniazid for latent tuberculosis infection. N Engl J Med 2011;365(23): 2155–66.

28. Menzies D, Adjobimey M, Ruslami R, et al. Four months of rifampin or nine months of isoniazid for latent tuberculosis in adults. N Engl J Med 2018; 379(5):440–53.

29. Sterling TR, Scott NA, Miro JM, et al. Three months of weekly rifapentine and isoniazid for treatment of Mycobacterium tuberculosis infection in HIV-coinfected persons. AIDS 2016;30(10): 1607–15.

30. Villarino ME, Scott NA, Weis SE, et al. Treatment for preventing tuberculosis in children and adolescents: a randomized clinical trial of a 3-month, 12-dose regimen of a combination of rifapentine and isoniazid. JAMA Pediatr 2015;169(3):247–55.

31. Subbaraman R, Nathavitharana RR, Satyanarayana S, et al. The tuberculosis cascade of care in India's public sector: a systematic review and meta-analysis. PLoS Med 2016;13(10):e1002149.

32. The Stop TB Partnership. The paradigm shift. The Global Plan to End TB. Stop TB Partnership. Geneva, Switzerland. 2015.

Current Medical Management of Pulmonary Tuberculosis

Robert W. Belknap, MD[a,b,*]

KEYWORDS

- Pulmonary tuberculosis • TB diagnosis • TB treatment • Drug-susceptible TB • Drug-resistant TB

KEY POINTS

- Diagnosing pulmonary tuberculosis early requires recognizing the various symptoms and radiographic presentations of disease.
- Nucleic acid amplification tests are more sensitive and specific than sputum smears and are increasingly used.
- Isoniazid, rifampin, pyrazinamide, and ethambutol remain the first-line treatment of pulmonary tuberculosis worldwide.
- Newer and repurposed medications offer the potential to improve treatment outcomes for drug-resistant tuberculosis (eg, bedaquiline, delamanid, pretomanid, linezolid, moxifloxacin, levofloxacin, and clofazimine).
- Treatment of patients with comorbidities like HIV, renal failure, and liver disease is more complicated but can be managed.

INTRODUCTION

Tuberculosis (TB) has afflicted people for millennia and, unfortunately, despite effective treatment was the leading cause of death from an infection in 2016, killing 1.7 million people globally.[1,2] TB is also a common cause of disease and death among people living with HIV. Recent estimates suggest that one-quarter of the world's population is infected with TB and more than 10 million people develop active disease each year.[1,3] Infection occurs primarily through airborne transmission and usually requires prolonged exposure to a person with pulmonary TB. The initial infection results in spread of organisms from the lungs to local lymph nodes followed by dissemination through the blood. Approximately 5% of people develop progressive disease after initial infection and this is more common in young children and people with immunosuppression. For most, their immune system controls the infection, ultimately forming granulomas without ever being symptomatic.

TB can remain hidden in individuals for decades before progressing to cause clinical disease. Reactivation may be associated with other conditions that weaken the immune system, such as HIV or diabetes, but often occurs in otherwise healthy people. When it occurs, reactivation TB involves the lungs in approximately 75% of people.[1,4] Those with pulmonary TB are then able to spread it to others, perpetuating the cycle of infection that leads to disease. Early diagnosis and treatment of pulmonary TB help minimize TB transmission and are an important strategy for decreasing the global TB burden. Untreated, smear-positive pulmonary TB has a

---

Disclosure: The author has nothing to disclose.
[a] Denver Metro Tuberculosis Program, Denver Health and Hospital Authority, 605 Bannock, Denver, CO 80204, USA; [b] Division of Infectious Diseases, Department of Medicine, University of Colorado Denver Anschutz Medical Campus, 12700 East 18th Avenue, RC2, Aurora, CO 80045, USA
* Denver Metro Tuberculosis Program, 605 Bannock, Denver, CO 80204.
E-mail address: robert.belknap@dhha.org

Thorac Surg Clin 29 (2019) 27–35
https://doi.org/10.1016/j.thorsurg.2018.09.004
1547-4127/19/© 2018 Elsevier Inc. All rights reserved.

10-year mortality of 70%.[5] Late diagnoses also result in permanent lung damage for many patients.[6]

DIAGNOSIS
Risk and Symptoms

TB disease first requires infection, which usually occurs after prolonged exposure to someone with active pulmonary TB. Known close contact to a person with pulmonary TB is the greatest risk but is uncommon. Most people do not know when they were exposed and infected so being born or living in a TB-endemic country is the most common risk. Currently that includes most countries, with the exceptions of Western and Northern Europe, the United States, Canada, Australia, New Zealand, and Japan. Even within those countries, individual risk may vary by location and demographic factors, such as homelessness.

The first step in diagnosing pulmonary TB requires having suspicion for disease. Delays in diagnosis are common because the symptoms are nonspecific. Unlike most infectious diseases that either resolve or get progressively worse, TB may wax and wane even without treatment. As a result, patients may not recognize their symptoms as the same illness, resulting in delays presenting for care. TB should be considered in patients who present with a subacute illness, particularly if they have lived in a country where TB is endemic. People with risk for TB infection and who have certain other medical conditions are at higher risk for developing disease. Those at greatest risk are people living with HIV, adult and child contacts of pulmonary TB, patients initiating anti–tumor necrosis factor alpha treatment, patients receiving dialysis, patients receiving organ or hematologic transplantation, and patients with silicosis. People with diabetes are also at higher risk than the general public, and diabetes is one of the most common comorbidities associated with active TB.[7] Importantly, most people who develop active TB do not have one of these associated conditions. Typical symptoms for pulmonary TB include

- Cough greater than 3 weeks that is typically productive of sputum, worsens over time, and may be associated with hemoptysis
- Dyspnea
- Fever
- Night sweats
- Weight loss
- Chest pain (with pleural disease)

Imaging

Chest imaging should be done for anyone suspected of having pulmonary TB. A posteroanterior chest radiograph is generally sufficient for evaluating adults and adolescents. A lateral chest radiograph is helpful in younger children to look for hilar adenopathy and retrocardiac infiltrates. Classically described radiographic findings are upper lobe fibronodular opacities with or without cavitation (**Fig. 1**). Miliary TB appears as small nodules scattered diffusely throughout both lungs (**Fig. 2**). TB can present with consolidations that look radiographically similar to bacterial pneumonia. Empiric antibiotics for bacterial infection can cause a delayed TB diagnosis. This is particularly true when fluoroquinolones are prescribed because they have excellent activity against most strains. Other radiographic presentations of pulmonary TB include solitary or multiple nodules, masses, adenopathy (**Fig. 3**), and pleural effusion.

CT scans of the chest show the extent of disease in greater detail than plain radiographs but are rarely needed for the diagnosis or management of TB. When pulmonary TB is suspected, CT scans should be deferred while collecting respiratory specimens for acid-fast bacilli (AFB). CT scans may be beneficial when respiratory specimens are initially negative or other diagnoses are considered likely. The chest CT findings in patients with active TB vary but may include tree-in-bud or ground-glass opacities, fibrosis, nodules, cavitation, pleural effusions, and hilar or mediastinal adenopathy.[8]

PET scans have been used in research studies to better understand the pathophysiology of TB.[9,10] PET scans have also been suggested as a tool for diagnosing TB and monitoring response to therapy.[11] They are not able to differentiate TB from malignancy very well but could be helpful in

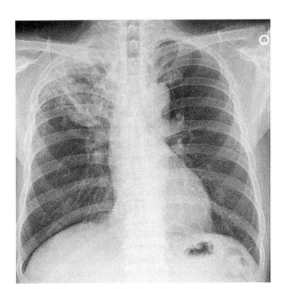

Fig. 1. Right upper lobe fibrotic opacities.

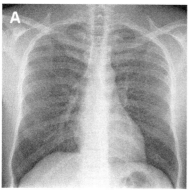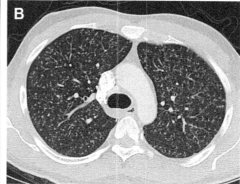

Fig. 2. (*A*) Miliary TB on chest radiograph. (*B*) Miliary TB on CT.

identifying active lesions for biopsy. Cost and access are likely to remain major barriers to routine use.

Microbiologic Specimens

Sputum samples are the hallmark for diagnosing pulmonary TB and AFB smears remain the initial test. The sensitivity of AFB smears increases with serial specimens from approximately 54% with 1 specimen, 65% with 2 specimens, and up to 70% with 3 specimens.[12] The quality of the sputum is generally more important than the timing although an early morning sputa is more sensitive than a single spot specimen.[13] Early morning sputa may also be easier to collect for patients with minimal symptoms. Sputum collection every 6 hours to 8 hours, particularly in hospitalized patients, facilitates more rapid diagnosis and minimizes the time in isolation for people without TB.

Bronchoscopy is not generally needed to diagnose pulmonary TB.[14] Sputum induction is as effective, less expensive than, and less invasive for patients who are unable to expectorate sputum. Bronchoscopy should be considered for patients who fail sputum induction or when an alternative diagnosis is considered likely. In patients with miliary disease who undergo bronchoscopy, bronchial brushings or transbronchial biopsy are more sensitive than bronchoalveolar lavage.[12]

Nucleic acid amplification tests (NAATs) are more sensitive and specific than AFB smears for diagnosing TB. The GeneXpert (Cepheid, USA) requires minimal specimen processing and laboratory expertise that have made it feasible to use in resource limited settings. A single GeneXpert can detect 97% of sputum smear positive TB and nearly 60% of smear-negative, culture-positive disease whereas a second test increases the sensitivity to 100% and 70%, respectively.[15] Based on these results, GeneXpert was approved in the United States for removing hospitalized patients with negative results from respiratory isolation. Many NAATs are also able to detect resistance mutations, allowing a shorter time to

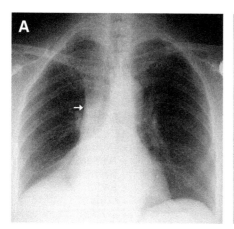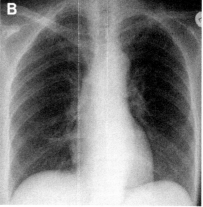

Fig. 3. (*A*) Paratracheal adenopathy *(arrow)* in a patient with HIV. (*B*) Resolution of adenopathy with treatment.

starting effective treatment. Susceptibility and resistance should still be confirmed with culture whenever possible.

Pleural TB typically presents with a unilateral, exudative effusion that is lymphocyte predominant. AFB smears and cultures from pleural fluid generally detect less than 50% of active TB.[12] Pleural biopsy with tissue sent for pathology and cultures is the best method for definitively diagnosing pleural TB. Closed needle biopsy is effective in most patients whereas thoracoscopic biopsy for histopathology and culture is diagnostic in nearly 100% of cases. Pleural fluid adenosine deaminase has moderate sensitivity and specificity and may be helpful in settings where pleural biopsy is not feasible.[16]

Culture remains the gold standard for diagnosing TB and should be done whenever possible. Growing TB allows for a definitive diagnosis and testing for drug susceptibility. Unfortunately, cultures are rarely done for patients with newly diagnosed TB in resource limited settings. The cost and complexity of maintaining laboratory capacity have prevented widespread use so cultures are generally limited to those with treatment failure or relapse. Liquid cultures provide the shortest time to growth and first-line susceptibility testing. Solid media are beneficial for isolating TB when there is contamination and testing susceptibility to second-line drugs when needed.

Tuberculin Skin Test and Interferon-Gamma Release Assays

The tuberculin skin test and interferon-gamma release assays (IGRAs) are immunologic tests for diagnosing TB infection. The 2 commercially available IGRAs are QuantiFERON-TB (Qiagen, Germany) and T-SPOT.TB (Oxford Immunotec, United Kingdom). These tests should never be used to rule out TB and have a limited role in diagnosing active disease. The tuberculin skin test misses up to 30% of people with active TB whereas the IGRAs miss approximately 10% to 15%.[17] They may be helpful when trying to decide whether to treat someone empirically for TB who otherwise has negative AFB smears or NAATs while waiting for cultures. These decisions are best made in consultation with the local public health providers who can evaluate the public health risk of delaying treatment.

Other Testing

Additional testing is important for the management of patients with suspected or confirmed TB but does not aid in the diagnosis. All patients with suspected TB should be tested for HIV. Other laboratory tests that are important include a complete blood cell count, hepatic function panel, and creatinine. Tests done within the prior few months are usually sufficient. Baseline visual acuity and color vision should be documented and monitored monthly for people receiving ethambutol (EMB). Additional testing and monitoring may be needed in patients with drug-resistant TB depending on the medications used.

TREATMENT
Drug-Susceptible Tuberculosis

Standard first-line treatment of pulmonary TB consists of isoniazid (INH), rifampin (RIF),

Table 1
Medications for drug-susceptible tuberculosis

Drug	Common or Severe Adverse Effects
INH	• Headache • Fatigue • Nausea/anorexia/abdominal pain • Drug-induced hepatitis • Rash • Peripheral neuropathy
RIF	• Drug-drug interactions • Red/orange discoloration of body fluids • Rash • Nausea/anorexia/abdominal pain • Flulike illness/hypersensitivity • Drug-induced hepatitis • Acute renal failure • Anemia/thrombocytopenia
PZA	• Nausea/anorexia/abdominal pain • Drug-induced hepatitis • Rash/acute flushing • Join pain • Elevated uric acid
EMB	• Visual impairment/optic neuritis
Levofloxacin	• Headache/insomnia • Nausea/anorexia/abdominal pain • Rash • QT prolongation • Tendonitis/tendon rupture
Moxofloxacin	• Headache/insomnia • Nausea/anorexia/abdominal pain • Rash • QT prolongation • Tendonitis/tendon rupture • Drug-induced hepatitis

pyrazinamide (PZA), and EMB.[18,19] **Table 1** lists the common and potential severe adverse effects from these medications. With this combination, INH has the best early bactericidal activity whereas RIF is necessary to cure TB in the shortest time. PZA is effective against minimally active organisms and inclusion in the first 2 months facilitates cure with a 6-month course. EMB is the least active in this combination but is protective against acquired resistance when treatment is started without knowing the susceptibilities. This combination of medications is given for 2 months in the initial phase of TB treatment. With fully susceptible TB, EMB is not needed and the initial 2 months of treatment can be with INH, RIF, and PZA alone.

The continuation phase for drug-susceptible TB is INH and RIF. The usual duration is 4 months to complete 6 months of total treatment. There is no test to determine when a person has been cured, so the goal of treatment is to achieve a low risk for relapse (generally <5%). Factors known to be associated with higher relapse rates are cavitation, positive sputum culture after 2 months of treatment, and being underweight at the start and failing to gain weight during treatment.[20,21] A common approach is to extend treatment by 3 months (9 months total) for patients with 1 or more risks for relapse. Similarly, patients whose TB is resistant to PZA or who are cannot complete 2 months of that medication can be treated with a 9-month course of INH and RIF.[18]

Isoniazid Resistance or Intolerance

When INH cannot be given because of resistance or intolerance, a fluoroquinolone (moxifloxacin or levofloxacin) is often given in combination with RIF, PZA, and EMB for the initial phase. For the continuation phase, the options are to continue treatment with RIF, PZA, or EMB or to continue the fluoroquinolone and RIF with or without EMB.[18] The combination of RIF, PZA, and EMB throughout is as effective as treatment with INH and RIF for drug-susceptible TB but may not be well tolerated.[22] A retrospective evaluation of patients with INH-resistant TB found that patients who received a fluoroquinolone in combination with RIF and EMB had good outcomes.[23] A recent study evaluated the role of moxifloxacin in different experimental arms with a primary goal of shortening treatment to 4 months. One experimental arm received moxifloxacin, RIF, PZA, and EMB daily for 2 months followed by once-weekly moxifloxacin and rifapentine for 4 months.[24] The 4-month treatment arms were inferior to the standard 6-month daily regimen but the experimental arm with the once-weekly continuation phase for

4 months was as effective as the standard regimen. Potential adverse effects from levofloxacin and moxifloxacin are listed in **Table 1**.

Multidrug-Resistant and Extensively Drug-Resistant Tuberculosis

Multidrug-resistant (MDR) TB is defined as resistance to INH and RIF with or without resistance to other drugs. Empiric treatment should include 4 to 6 drugs that are likely to be active.[25,26] Fluoroquinolones and injectable drugs have been the cornerstone of treatment of MDR TB. Moxifloxacin is often chosen over levofloxacin based on in vitro data but both drugs are effective.[27] All oral regimens using newer drugs are being evaluated for efficacy and safety and may replace older regimens that include an injectable drug for many months.[28–30] Treatment durations had typically been 18 months to 24 months but a 9-month regimen has shown promise and shorter durations using novel combinations are being evaluated.[31–33]

Extensively drug-resistant (XDR) TB is resistant to INH and RIF plus fluoroquinolones and at least 1 second-line injectable drug (amikacin, kanamycin, or capreomycin).[19,26] The basic principles are the same as treating MDR TB. Treatment of XDR TB should be done in consultation with an expert in treating drug-resistant TB. A general principle is to include 5 to 6 drugs likely to have activity. PZA may be included despite phenotypic resistance with the hope that it might retain some activity against the minimally active organisms. Some providers also use high doses of moxifloxacin and/or INH when low-level resistance to these drugs is found or when there are few other options. Linezolid has become an important component of treatment regimens for both MDR TB and XDR TB.[34,35] Although the optimal dose is unknown, observational studies giving one-half the usual daily dose for bacterial infections seems effective and has less toxicity. Bedaquiline is another newer drug that is becoming increasingly important for treating drug-resistant TB.[36] Other new and repurposed medications that are showing efficacy include delamanid, pretomanid, and clofazimine.[30]

MONITORING TREATMENT

Ensuring adherence to treatment is important to minimize the risk of failure, acquired drug resistance, and TB transmission. Directly observed therapy (DOT) maximizes treatment completion, allows close monitoring for drug-related side effects, and is the standard of care for patients with pulmonary TB. Intermittent dosing strategies were developed to make DOT easier for patients and providers. Although outcomes with intermittent dosing were generally comparable to daily therapy, recent meta-analyses have shown higher rates of relapse including in patients with HIV.[37–39] Therefore, current guidelines recommend daily therapy unless intermittent therapy is the only feasible option.[18,19] Because daily DOT is difficult and costly for patients and programs, digital technology is increasingly used as a more affordable and patient-centered approach to treatment monitoring.[40–42] Some technologies allow patients and health care personnel to interact in real time.[40,41] Others allow patients to record a video of themselves taking the medications at a time they prefer. The video is then uploaded to a secure server and can be viewed by TB program staff during normal business hours.[42] Studies evaluating video DOT, either real-time or recorded, have found that adherence is comparable to in-person DOT with high levels of patient satisfaction.[42]

Patients are usually seen monthly at in-clinic visits to monitor their response to treatment and assess for drug-related toxicity. Visual acuity and color vision should be checked for patients taking EMB. Sputum cultures should be collected each month until there are 2 consecutive specimens that are negative. NAATs are not recommended at this time for monitoring response to treatment or suspected failure or relapse. These tests may detect TB DNA for months or even years after effective treatment in patients who are otherwise clinically well and have negative cultures.[43]

Laboratory monitoring for toxicity is not routinely needed. Liver function tests should be checked at least monthly in patients with known liver disease or baseline abnormalities. They should also be checked immediately in anyone who develops nausea, vomiting, abdominal pain, loss of appetite, or jaundice. Other laboratory tests should be done as needed based on symptoms or other medical conditions.

SPECIAL CIRCUMSTANCES
Tuberculosis and HIV

The approach to treating TB in people living with HIV is similar to treatment of HIV-negative individuals.[44] Relapse rates after 6 months of treatment of drug-susceptible pulmonary TB in people receiving treatment of HIV are low and comparable to people without HIV.[45] In individuals who are not started on antiretroviral therapy (ART) and are highly immunocompromised, extending treatment to 9 months may be beneficial.[18,46] The most important consideration is often the drug-drug interactions with RIF. Rifabutin may be needed to replace RIF with many ART combinations.

The timing of HIV treatment in people with pulmonary TB has been studied in several randomized trials. These studies showed that survival was higher in people with CD4 counts less than 50 cells/μL who started ART within 2 weeks of TB treatment. The exception is people with concomitant central nervous system disease because they are at high risk for immune reconstitution inflammatory syndrome (IRIS). The optimal timing to start ART in these individuals is unclear.[47] Patients with CD4 counts greater than 50 cells/μL can delay ART if needed but ideally should start within the first 2 months. The highest risk for IRIS is in the first 4 weeks to 12 weeks after starting ART.[48,49] ART can usually be continued in people experiencing IRIS. Corticosteroids may be beneficial in people with central nervous system disease or severe IRIS.[50]

Renal Disease

Patients with end-stage renal disease are at increased risk for TB and for poor outcomes from disease.[51] PZA and EMB are cleared by the kidneys and the doses must be adjusted when creatinine clearance is less than 30 mL/min. The recommendation is to give the usual daily dose 3 times per week after hemodialysis.[18] INH and RIF are metabolized by the liver so do not need to be adjusted. For patients treated with a fluoroquinolone, levofloxacin is cleared renally and can be dosed intermittently when the creatinine clearance is less than 50 mL/min. Moxifloxacin is cleared by the liver so can be given without dose adjustment.

Liver Disease

Patients with liver disease are also at risk for complications due to TB and TB treatment. INH, RIF, and PZA can all cause drug-induced liver injury. Reports suggest that PZA and INH are associated with more liver toxicity than RIF. RIF should be suspected when the total bilirubin and alkaline phosphatase are elevated out of proportion to the transaminases. Nevertheless, RIF is commonly tried without the other drugs after the liver function tests improve regardless of the pattern because it is the most effective drug for curing TB with the shortest treatment duration.

Optimal dosing of INH and RIF in patients with chronic liver disease is unknown and the choice of treatment depends on the degree of functional impairment. Patients with chronic liver disease without cirrhosis and whose baseline transaminases are less than 3 times the upper limit of normal can often be treated with standard therapy and close monitoring. PZA may be avoided in patients with moderate liver disease or higher risk of hepatotoxicity. Moxifloxacin is cleared by the liver and has rarely been associated with hepatotoxicity so levofloxacin may be preferred.

In patients with advanced liver disease, choosing a safe regimen can be difficult. Levofloxacin, EMB, and injectable medications are generally safe. RIF is often included with close clinical and laboratory monitoring given its importance for curing TB. Cycloserine, linezolid, and clofazimine are other TB treatments that have a low risk for hepatotoxicity but should be considered carefully given their potential nonhepatic toxicity.

Adjunctive Steroids and Tumor Necrosis Factor α Inhibitors

Active TB can cause severe inflammation at the site of disease that may worsen after starting TB treatment. This acute worsening has been termed a paradoxical reaction and is clinically similar to IRIS in people with HIV after starting ART. Depending on the site and extent of TB disease, these reactions can be severe and even life threatening. Systemic steroids have been used successfully to treat and prevent the complications of TB IRIS, as discussed previously.[50] In patients with TB meningitis, steroids have been shown to decrease the risk of death and are recommended as adjunctive therapy tapered over 6 weeks to 8 weeks.[52,53] Steroid therapy was commonly used in patients with TB pericarditis but a recent randomized controlled trial showed no benefit and it is no longer recommended by the US guidelines.[18,54] Adjunctive steroids have been used sporadically to treat severe pulmonary or miliary disease but its exact role in these forms of disease has not been established. Case reports have described using tumor necrosis factor α inhibitors to treat severe TB IRIS that was unresponsive to steroids and warrants further study.[55,56]

SUMMARY

Pulmonary TB remains a common disease globally and is usually a subacute illness. The primary strategy for diagnosing TB in high-burden, low-resource settings is through passive case finding that involves evaluating people who present for care due to symptoms. Lack of easy access to health care, stigma associated with TB, and fear of not being able to work often prevent people from seeking care early. Delays lead to progressive disease, permanent lung damage, and lifelong disability or death. Delays also increase the risk of transmission to others. Addressing the system-level, social, and financial barriers to seeking care are important to decreasing morbidity and mortality from pulmonary TB. Active case finding

by identifying and evaluating those at risk but with minimal or no symptoms is effective for diagnosing TB earlier but requires more resources.

The biggest advance in diagnostic testing has been with the NAATs that are more accurate than AFB smears for diagnosing pulmonary TB. The GeneXpert Omni is battery operated so can be used outside of a laboratory. This moves the technology closer to being a point-of-care test for rapid TB diagnosis. Continued improvements that minimize the need for specimen processing and decrease the cost are still needed.

Drug-susceptible pulmonary TB is curable but requires a combination of medications and a lengthy treatment course that has not changed in approximately 40 years. Increasing prevalence and severity of resistant TB threaten to reverse the recent declines in the global TB burden. DOT remains the standard of care for treating pulmonary TB to minimize the risks of acquired drug resistance and ongoing community transmission. Digital technologies offer a more patient-centered alternative to in-person DOT for monitoring adherence. New and repurposed drugs are providing minimal improvement in treating MDR TB and XDR TB. Outcomes are still unacceptably poor and treatment remains difficult and costly for patients and health care providers. Progress toward reducing the global burden of TB will continue to be slow without better diagnostic tools and medications that are well tolerated, safe, and effective, with a shorter duration than current treatment.

REFERENCES

1. World Health Organization. Global tuberculosis report. Geneva (Switzerland): WHO; 2017.
2. Zink AR, Sola C, Reischl U, et al. Characterization of Mycobacterium tuberculosis complex DNAs from Egyptian mummies by spoligotyping. J Clin Microbiol 2003;41:359–67.
3. Houben RM, Dodd PJ. The global burden of latent tuberculosis infection: a re-estimation using mathematical modelling. PLoS Med 2016;13:e1002152.
4. Stewart RJ, Isang CA, Pratt RH, et al. Tuberculosis — United States, 2017. MMWR Morb Mortal Wkly Rep 2018;67:317–23.
5. Tiemersma EW, van der Werf MJ, Borgdorff MW, et al. Natural history of tuberculosis: duration and fatality of untreated pulmonary tuberculosis in HIV negative patients: a systematic review. PLoS One 2011;6:e17601.
6. Ravimohan S, Kornfeld H, Weissman D, et al. Tuberculosis and lung damage: from epidemiology to pathophysiology. Eur Respir Rev 2018;27 [pii:170077].
7. Harries AD, Satyanarayana S, Kumar AM, et al. Epidemiology and interaction of diabetes mellitus

and tuberculosis and challenges for care: a review. Public Health Action 2013;3:S3–9.

8. Daley C, Gotway M, Jasmer R. Radiographic manifestations of tuberculosis. 2011. Available at: http://www.currytbcenter.ucsf.edu/topics-interest/tb-radiology. Accessed October 7, 2018.

9. Coleman MT, Chen RY, Lee M, et al. PET/CT imaging reveals a therapeutic response to oxazolidinones in macaques and humans with tuberculosis. Sci Transl Med 2014;6:265ra167.

10. Lin PL, Maiello P, Gideon HP, et al. PET CT identifies reactivation risk in cynomolgus macaques with latent M. tuberculosis. PLoS Pathog 2016;12: e1005739.

11. Vorster M, Sathekge MM, Bomanji J. Advances in imaging of tuberculosis: the role of (1)(8)F-FDG PET and PET/CT. Curr Opin Pulm Med 2014;20: 287–93.

12. Lewinsohn DM, Leonard MK, LoBue PA, et al. Official American Thoracic Society/Infectious Diseases Society of America/Centers for Disease Control and Prevention clinical practice guidelines: diagnosis of tuberculosis in adults and children. Clin Infect Dis 2017;64:e1–33.

13. Mase SR, Ramsay A, Ng V, et al. Yield of serial sputum specimen examinations in the diagnosis of pulmonary tuberculosis: a systematic review. Int J Tuberc Lung Dis 2007;11:485–95.

14. Brown M, Varia H, Bassett P, et al. Prospective study of sputum induction, gastric washing, and bronchoalveolar lavage for the diagnosis of pulmonary tuberculosis in patients who are unable to expectorate. Clin Infect Dis 2007;44:1415–20.

15. Luetkemeyer AF, Firnhaber C, Kendall MA, et al, AIDS Clinical Trials Group A5295 and Tuberculosis Trials Consortium Study 34 Teams. Evaluation of Xpert MTB/RIF versus AFB smear and culture to identify pulmonary tuberculosis in patients with suspected tuberculosis from low and higher prevalence settings. Clin Infect Dis 2016;62:1081–8.

16. Gui X, Xiao H. Diagnosis of tuberculosis pleurisy with adenosine deaminase (ADA): a systematic review and meta-analysis. Int J Clin Exp Med 2014;7: 3126–35.

17. Diel R, Loddenkemper R, Nienhaus A. Evidence-based comparison of commercial interferon-gamma release assays for detecting active TB: a metaanalysis. Chest 2010;137:952–68.

18. Nahid P, Dorman SE, Alipanah N, et al. Official American Thoracic Society/Centers for Disease Control and Prevention/Infectious Diseases Society of America clinical practice guidelines: treatment of drug-susceptible tuberculosis. Clin Infect Dis 2016;63: e147–95.

19. World Health Organization. Guidelines for treatment of drug-susceptible tuberculosis and patient care, 2017 update. Geneva (Switzerland): WHO; 2017.

20. Tuberculosis Trials Consortium. Once-weekly rifapentine and isoniazid versus twice-weekly rifampin and isoniazid in the continuation phase of therapy for drug-susceptible pulmonary tuberculosis: a prospective, randomized clinical trial among HIV-negative persons. Lancet 2002;360:528–34.

21. Khan A, Sterling TR, Reves R, et al. Lack of weight gain and relapse risk in a large tuberculosis treatment trial. Am J Respir Crit Care Med 2006;174:344–8.

22. Gegia M, Winters N, Benedetti A, et al. Treatment of isoniazid-resistant tuberculosis with first-line drugs: a systematic review and meta-analysis. Lancet Infect Dis 2017;17:223–34.

23. Schechter MC, Bizune D, Kagei M, et al. Time to sputum culture conversion and treatment outcomes among patients with isoniazid-resistant tuberculosis in Atlanta, Georgia. Clin Infect Dis 2017;65:1862–71.

24. Jindani A, Harrison TS, Nunn AJ, et al. High-dose rifapentine with moxifloxacin for pulmonary tuberculosis. N Engl J Med 2014;371:1599–608.

25. World Health Organization. WHO treatment guidelines for drug resistant tuberculosis. Geneva (Switzerland): WHO; 2016.

26. Drug-Resistant Tuberculosis, a survival guide for clinicians 3rd edition. 2016. Available at: http://www.currytbcenter.ucsf.edu/products/view/drug-resistant-tuberculosis-survival-guide-clinicians-3rd-edition. Accessed October 7, 2018.

27. Kang YA, Shim TS, Koh WJ, et al. Choice between levofloxacin and moxifloxacin and multidrug-resistant tuberculosis treatment outcomes. Ann Am Thorac Soc 2016;13:364–70.

28. Dawson R, Diacon AH, Everitt D, et al. Efficiency and safety of the combination of moxifloxacin, pretomanid (PA-824), and pyrazinamide during the first 8 weeks of antituberculosis treatment: a phase 2b, open-label, partly randomised trial in patients with drug-susceptible or drug-resistant pulmonary tuberculosis. Lancet 2015;385:1738–47.

29. Reuter A, Tisile P, von Delft D, et al. The devil we know: is the use of injectable agents for the treatment of MDR-TB justified? Int J Tuberc Lung Dis 2017;21:1114–26.

30. Chang KC, Nuermberger E, Sotgiu G, et al. New drugs and regimens for tuberculosis. Respirology 2018. https://doi.org/10.1111/resp.13345.

31. Van Deun A, Maug AK, Salim MA, et al. Short, highly effective, and inexpensive standardized treatment of multidrug-resistant tuberculosis. Am J Respir Crit Care Med 2010;182:684–92.

32. Aung KJ, Van Deun A, Declercq E, et al. Successful '9-month Bangladesh regimen' for multidrug-resistant tuberculosis among over 500 consecutive patients. Int J Tuberc Lung Dis 2014;18:1180–7.

33. Sotgiu G, Tiberi S, Centis R, et al. Applicability of the shorter 'Bangladesh regimen' in high multidrug-resistant tuberculosis settings. Int J Infect Dis 2017;56:190–3.

34. Berry C, Yates TA, Seddon JA, et al. Efficacy, safety and tolerability of linezolid for the treatment of XDR-TB: a study in China. Eur Respir J 2016;47:1591–2.

35. Agyeman AA, Ofori-Asenso R. Efficacy and safety profile of linezolid in the treatment of multidrug-resistant (MDR) and extensively drug-resistant (XDR) tuberculosis: a systematic review and meta-analysis. Ann Clin Microbiol Antimicrob 2016;15:41.

36. Borisov SE, Dheda K, Enwerem M, et al. Effectiveness and safety of bedaquiline-containing regimens in the treatment of MDR- and XDR-TB: a multicentre study. Eur Respir J 2017;49 [pii:1700387].

37. Burman W, Benator D, Vernon A, et al. Acquired rifamycin resistance with twice-weekly treatment of HIV-related tuberculosis. Am J Respir Crit Care Med 2006;173:350–6.

38. Johnston JC, Campbell JR, Menzies D. Effect of intermittency on treatment outcomes in pulmonary tuberculosis: an updated systematic review and metaanalysis. Clin Infect Dis 2017;64:1211–20.

39. Gopalan N, Santhanakrishnan RK, Palaniappan AN, et al. Daily vs intermittent antituberculosis therapy for pulmonary tuberculosis in patients with hiv: a randomized clinical trial. JAMA Intern Med 2018;178: 485–93.

40. DeMaio J, Schwartz L, Cooley P, et al. The application of telemedicine technology to a directly observed therapy program for tuberculosis: a pilot project. Clin Infect Dis 2001;33:2082–4.

41. Krueger K, Ruby D, Cooley P, et al. Videophone utilization as an alternative to directly observed therapy for tuberculosis. Int J Tuberc Lung Dis 2010; 14:779–81.

42. Garfein RS, Collins K, Munoz F, et al. Feasibility of tuberculosis treatment monitoring by video directly observed therapy: a binational pilot study. Int J Tuberc Lung Dis 2015;19:1057–64.

43. Theron G, Venter R, Smith L, et al. False-positive Xpert MTB/RIF results in retested patients with previous tuberculosis: frequency, profile, and prospective clinical outcomes. J Clin Microbiol 2018;56(3). e01696-17.

44. Haas MK, Daley CL. Mycobacterial lung disease complicating HIV infection. Semin Respir Crit Care Med 2016;37:230–42.

45. Mfinanga SG, Kirenga BJ, Chanda DM, et al. Early versus delayed initiation of highly active antiretroviral therapy for HIV-positive adults with newly diagnosed pulmonary tuberculosis (TB-HAART): a prospective, international, randomised, placebo-controlled trial. Lancet Infect Dis 2014;14: 563–71.

46. Nahid P, Gonzalez LC, Rudoy I, et al. Treatment outcomes of patients with HIV and tuberculosis. Am J Respir Crit Care Med 2007;175:1199–206.

47. Torok ME, Yen NT, Chau TT, et al. Timing of initiation of antiretroviral therapy in human immunodeficiency virus (HIV)–associated tuberculous meningitis. Clin Infect Dis 2011;52:1374–83.

48. Naidoo K, Yende-Zuma N, Padayatchi N, et al. The immune reconstitution inflammatory syndrome after antiretroviral therapy initiation in patients with tuberculosis: findings from the SAPiT trial. Ann Intern Med 2012;157:313–24.

49. Lawn SD, Myer L, Bekker LG, et al. Tuberculosis-associated immune reconstitution disease: incidence, risk factors and impact in an antiretroviral treatment service in South Africa. AIDS 2007;21: 335–41.

50. Meintjes G, Wilkinson RJ, Morroni C, et al. Randomized placebo-controlled trial of prednisone for paradoxical tuberculosis-associated immune reconstitution inflammatory syndrome. AIDS 2010;24: 2381–90.

51. Baghaei P, Marjani M, Tabarsi P, et al. Impact of chronic renal failure on anti-tuberculosis treatment outcomes. Int J Tuberc Lung Dis 2014;18:352–6.

52. Critchley JA, Young F, Orton L, et al. Corticosteroids for prevention of mortality in people with tuberculosis: a systematic review and meta-analysis. Lancet Infect Dis 2013;13:223–37.

53. Prasad K, Singh MB, Ryan H. Corticosteroids for managing tuberculous meningitis. Cochrane Database Syst Rev 2016;(4):CD002244.

54. Mayosi BM, Ntsekhe M, Bosch J, et al. Prednisolone and Mycobacterium indicus pranii in tuberculous pericarditis. N Engl J Med 2014;371:1121–30.

55. Wallis RS, van Vuuren C, Potgieter S. Adalimumab treatment of life-threatening tuberculosis. Clin Infect Dis 2009;48:1429–32.

56. Hsu DC, Faldetta KF, Pei L, et al. A paradoxical treatment for a paradoxical condition: infliximab use in three cases of mycobacterial IRIS. Clin Infect Dis 2016;62:258–61.

Surgical Resection in the Treatment of Pulmonary Tuberculosis

Piotr K. Yablonskii, MD, PhD[a,b], Grigorii G. Kudriashov, MD[a,*],
Armen O. Avetisyan, MD, PhD[a]

KEYWORDS

- Pulmonary resection for TB • Surgical treatment of tuberculosis • Minimally invasive surgery

KEY POINTS

- Surgical resection is an efficient and safe method in complex treatment of pulmonary tuberculosis.
- Pulmonary resection should be performed for unilateral and some variants of bilateral localized tuberculosis.
- Outcome of surgical treatment directly depends on the quality of surgery and adequacy of perioperative antituberculosis chemotherapy.
- Early rehabilitation of patients and early beginning of chemotherapy after surgery are necessary.
- A minimally invasive approach is preferable.

INTRODUCTION

Lung resections have been always the shortest way of removal of the affected zone of the lung with the hope of future recovery of tuberculosis (TB) patients. Nevertheless the successes in TB treatment of the second half of the twentieth century led to a complete abandonment of surgery as a method of TB treatment. It happened mostly in the countries of Western Europe, in the United States, and in Canada. At the same time, pulmonary resection continued to be performed not only for cavitary TB and sequelae of TB but also for tuberculomas; in cases of single foci of TB and even in calcifications it have been undertaken in the Eastern Europe, in the Russian Federation, and in the former Soviet republics. No evidence-based research regarding this approach for general population health improvement was published, although this large-scale work has allowed rescuing the traditions of the best surgical schools and saving qualified staff.

Social cataclysms of the last decade of the twentieth century, impoverishment of entire countries and regions of the Middle East, human migration, weakening of the general culture of TB control, noncompliance with approved chemotherapy regimens, and often voluntaristic approach to the appointment of chemotherapy provoked an epidemic of multidrug-resistant (MDR)–extensively drug resistant (XDR) TB. All told, an almost complete stop of new drug development and insufficient results of medication treatment of such patients (with M-/XDR - TB) increased the interest in surgery in many countries recently.

The epidemic situation led the World Health Organization (WHO) to create a working group of the clinical practice guidelines for pulmonary TB. The group of experts worked out a consensus

Disclosure: The authors have nothing to disclose.
[a] St. Petersburg State Research Institute of Phthisiopulmonology, Ligovskiy Avenue, 2-4, Saint Petersburg 191036, Russia; [b] St. Petersburg State University, Universitetskaya Embankment, 13B, Saint Petersburg 199034, Russia
* Corresponding author.
E-mail address: dr.kudriashov.gg@yandex.com

Thorac Surg Clin 29 (2019) 37–46
https://doi.org/10.1016/j.thorsurg.2018.09.003
1547-4127/19/© 2018 Elsevier Inc. All rights reserved.

document that unified different surgical approaches in complex pulmonary TB treatment.[1,2]

As the authors have shown in a publication in 2016,[3] lung resections remain the most effective way for conversion of sputum smears. Subotic and colleagues discuss possibilities of resection surgery in pulmonary TB treatments. The indication for surgery is made for life saving, sometimes in emergency situations, and especially in cases of inefficiency of previous treatment.

When considering a lung resection, surgeons must be aware of all details of the disease in TB patient. Is the lesion localized in 1 lobe, in 1 segment, or in 1 lung? Is it a bilateral TB or disseminated TB? Does the patient suffer from diabetes or has the patient had a transplantation surgery or is taking immunosuppressants or gene-modified drugs?

The authors do not discuss the different lung resections to verify a diagnosis. The authors discuss radical operations that offer a life chance for pulmonary TB patients in cases of adequate personalized TB chemotherapy and after a multidisciplinary approach to treatment of all concomitant diseases in a particular patient. The authors also describe the technical issues of lung resections and the place of minimally invasive and robot-assisted surgery in the treatment of pulmonary TB.

INDICATIONS FOR PULMONARY RESECTION IN TUBERCULOSIS CASES

Current indications for surgery (including first, pulmonary resection) were described by a working group of the WHO in a consensus document in 2014. There were 3 types of indications:

- Emergency (profuse lung hemorrhage and tension spontaneous pneumothorax), urgent (irreversible TB progression and recurrent hemoptysis that cannot be stopped by other treatment methods)
- Elective (localized forms of cavitary TB with continuous *Mycobacterium tuberculosis* [MTB] excretion confirmed by bacteriologic examination and after 4 months to 6 months of supervised anti-TB chemotherapy according to DST; MDR-/XDR-TB characterized by failure of anti-TB chemotherapy)
- Complications and sequelae of the TB process (including MDR-TB, XDR-TB)[1]

Most cases of TB require surgery according to elective indications. Surgery should be seriously considered when the disease is sufficiently localized to allow surgery; the remaining lung tissue around the resection margins is estimated to be free of TB; or a patient's surgical risk level is acceptable, with sufficient pulmonary reserve to tolerate the resection.[4]

The formation of cavities on the background of controlled chemotherapy, as a rule, is accompanied by the development of secondary drug-resistant MTB in most patients. Therefore, surgical resection of cavitary altered part of the lung in patients with pulmonary TB is not only a method of treatment but also an effective measure to prevent the spread of TB. The main condition for performing a pulmonary resection in such cases is an accurate conviction that the continuation of chemotherapy will fail. In sputum-negative patients, the decision to use the surgical resection should be taken no earlier than 4 months after the beginning of controlled chemotherapy. In patients with persistent bacterial excretion, it should not be earlier than after 6 months chemotherapy, according to the results of the drug susceptibility test of MTB. The main purpose of surgical pulmonary resection for cavitary TB is elimination of the source of MTB.[4]

The rate of treatment success after resection surgery for single-sided TB ranges between 75% and 98%. Unfortunately, patients with the most severe cases (eg, bilateral cavities or destroyed lung) who would benefit most from surgery cannot undergo such procedures due to high operative and postoperative morbidity and mortality. Surgery in such severe cases is also possible with a good result, but only in well-selected cases and after discussion of the surgical approach by a multidisciplinary team.[3]

Pulmonary Resection for Tuberculosis Complicated by Pulmonary Bleeding

Management of massive hemoptysis and timing of surgical intervention pose difficult problems. Mortality rate is 18% with surgery compared with a 75% rate in those treated conservatively. Emergency surgery should be reserved for those patients (1) who have adequate lung function, (2) in whom exact site of bleeding definitely defined, (3) and in whom there is continuing bleeding despite adequate measures taken. Emergency surgery performed for massive hemoptysis always has a higher risk than planned surgery. The complication rate is reported to increase with emergency pneumonectomy compared with emergency lobectomy (72% vs 52%). Generally accompanying dense pleural adhesions, presence of enlarged sticky lymph nodes, bronchiectasis, and broncholithiasis make the surgery complex and difficult.[5] The unsatisfactory results of emergency surgery for tuberculosis complicated by massive bleeding do not allow the use of this method everywhere. At the same time, endovascular embolization of the bronchial arteries and endobronchial valving can be recommended as a safety option for majority of patients.

PREOPERATIVE ASSESSMENT AND SELECTION OF PATIENTS FOR PULMONARY RESECTION

The patient is selected for pulmonary resection primarily when it is possible to remove the main source of infection. The remaining cases (bilateral TB, generalized TB infection etc.) should be discussed by a multidisciplinary team. Preoperative examination should include general and biochemical blood analysis, coagulogram, HIV testing, sputum smear microscopy for the detection of acid-fast bacilli, microbiological and molecular genetic studies for detection of mycobacteria of the TB complex and determination of drug sensitivity of the pathogen, standard chest radiography, chest CT, and fibrobronchoscopy.[4]

One classification for CT findings was proposed by Yi-Ting Yen and coauthors,[6] who investigated in a retrospective study the main signs that can influence the surgical tactic and surgical access for pulmonary TB. Image characteristics on chest CT scans were classified as bullae, pleural thickening, peribronchial lymph node calcification, tuberculoma, cavity, aspergilloma, atelectasis, and bronchiectasis, and graded according to the number of the lesions and degree of lobar involvement. As a result, authors calculated that multiple cavities, multiple aspergillomas, multilobar tuberculoma, extensive pleural thickening, and peribronchial lymph node calcification preclude video-assisted thoracoscopic surgery (VATS). It is reasonable to attempt a thoracoscopic approach in patients without these preoperative image characteristics.[6]

Functional examination of patients should include spirometry (for evaluation of vital capacity and forced expiratory volume in the first second of expiration [FEV$_1$]), ECG, and echocardiography. In patients with borderline pulmonary function testing results (FEV$_1$ <2.0 L) in the preoperative examination plan, perfusion lung scintigraphy and arterial gas analysis should be included. All patients with pulmonary TB who are referred for surgery (except in emergency situations) should have documented results of molecular genetic and/or microbiological studies, including a drug susceptibility test.

Comorbidity should also be carefully evaluated before surgery (Charlson comorbidity index for example). Attention should be paid to diabetes

and HIV infection, because this diseases may worsen the outcome of the surgery.

There are a few contraindications for pulmonary resection:

- Total cavitary disease of the both lungs, impairment of lung function (FEV$_1$ <1.5 L for lobectomy)
- Pulmonary heart failure of grades III–IV (New York Heart Association classification)
- Body mass index up to 40% to 50% of normal, severe comorbidities (decompensated diabetes mellitus)
- Exacerbation of peptic ulcer of stomach and duodenum, hepatic or renal insufficiency
- Active bronchial TB[4]

PERIOPERATIVE CARE

Standard anesthesiologic assessment includes general anesthesia with double-lumen intubation for better control of the bronchial secretion and the level of bronchial resection, single-pulmonary ventilation. Endoscopic control of endobronchial tube and bronchial stump is routine practice for pulmonary resection. All patients should be extubated on the operating table or in the ICU in the first hours after the operation. During the first postoperative day, cardiorespiratory system and correction of water-electrolyte balance, antibiotic prophylaxis, prophylaxis of thromboembolic complications, inhalation therapy, and respiratory gymnastics must be performed. Essential components of postoperative therapy are pain control, prevention of the arterial thromboembolism, treatment of comorbid diseases. The principal statement of the authors' clinic was in use of vacuum-aspiration drainage of the pleural cavity from the first hours after the operation.[7]

TECHNICAL ASPECTS OF SURGICAL RESECTIONS FOR PULMONARY TUBERCULOSIS

There are 4 basic types of resection surgery: wedge resection, anatomic segmentectomy, lobectomy/bilobectomy, and pneumonectomy.

Basic principles of pulmonary resections for tuberculosis include:

- "classical" technique of anatomical pulmonary resection with separate isolation and intersection of yhe hilar structures.
- careful isolation of lung from adhesions (sometimes in the extrapleural layer, if localization of cavity is superficially).

- careful isolation of hilar structures (calcified lymph nodes and hilar fibrosis may be causes of technical difficulties).
- sometimes procedures for reduce of the chest volume are necessary: transdiaphragmatic artificial pneumoperitoneum, intrapleural thoracoplasty (to improve the compliance of the lung and pleural cavity; also some surgeons use these methods to prevent the exacerbation of tuberculosis in the operated lung after surgery in patients with dissemination).

Sublobar Resection (Wedge Resection and Segmentectomy)

Sublobar resection makes up to 30% of all pulmonary resections for pulmonary TB and it may be anatomic or nonanatomic (wedge resection). Wedge resection is easy, but it can be used in a limited number of patients with residual TB lesions located under the visceral pleura. Wedge resection may be helpful also as additional step of polysegmental resections. Unrecognized TB foci entrapped with the stapler line during nonanatomic lung resections increase the risk of TB reactivation and contamination of the pleural cavity. A majority of indications for segmentectomy are tuberculomas and small cavities localized in the intersegmental boundaries between 2 segments. Segmentectomy for TB requires careful identification of the intersegmental plane and demarcation zone of the TB lesion. A probe with ventilation of the operated lung can help find the borders of a segment. One important "viewpoint" is division of the intersegmental plane following the intersegmental vein. Another method is to identify borders after closure of the "pulmonary vessels" and indocyanine green injection. Preoperative 3-D modeling of the segmental anatomy can also make performing segmentectomy easier. All of these methods were clearly described for lung cancer surgery, but it should be implemented for TB patients also.[1,4]

Lobectomy and Bilobectomy

Lobectomy and bilobectomy constitute up to 41.6% of all lung resections in some institutions. The indication for lobectomy is a tuberculous lesion located within the boundaries of a single lobe. To prevent any unintended opening of subpleural cavities, extrapleural resection should be used freely but limited to the areas with dense pleural adhesions. Sclerosed and calcified lymph nodes can be a cause of technical difficulties during the separation of hilar structures especially in cases with total damage of the lobe. Lymphadenectomy is not a mandatory element of surgery for TB. The removal of lymph nodes is justified to facilitate the dissection of the hilum elements. Bilobectomy for pulmonary TB is one of the rare type of surgery. Two articles show cases of pulmonary cavitary TB which were cured after bilobectomy with excellent postoperative follow-up.[1,4]

Combined and Rare Polysegmental Resection as Alternative to a Pneumonectomy

Anatomic lung resections in TB, which are more extensive than lobectomy, have special features connected with the prevalence of TB lesions, the severity of the specific process, and the need to perform intraoperative or postoperative prevention of exacerbation of the disease. This is the diverse group of patients and indications for polysegmental resections should be discussed by a multidisciplinary team only if there is no other medical options. This group of anatomic lung resections includes anatomic resections of different lobes: bilobectomy, bilobectomy plus segmentectomy, 1 lobe plus segmentectomy, and segmentectomy of the different lobes on the one side After such polysegmental resection, the patient may have from 3 to 6 healthy segments in the operated lung. All these variants of anatomic lung resections have their individual features as well as common features. Therefore, they represent 1 group, named combined anatomic lung resections. In the authors' clinic, they make up approximately 10% of the total number of operated patients.[8]

The choice in favor of combined anatomic lung resections or pneumonectomy always should be made by discuss with a multidisciplinary team; Conditions for the preservation of a part of the lung are no progression of pulmonary TB in the preoperative stage of treatment and relatively high blood flow (more than 15%) in the operated lung.[9]

The technique of polysegmental pulmonary resections is based on the principles of anatomical radicalism, with separate isolation of hilar structures and carefully division of the intersegmental plane with preservation of the venous outflow tracts. If surgical resection includes lobectomy plus segmentectomy, it should be more correct to begin with lobectomy and after that segmentectomy should be performed. In the absence of interlobar or intersegmental planes, the specimen should be removed in a "single block".

The difficulties of the polysegmental anatomical pulmonary resections related with a highly traumatic due to pleuropulmonary and hilar fibrotic process. These operations are accompanied with the sharp isolation of the lung in the extrapleural layer throughout the entire length or in a restricted area. There is a need for decortication of the lung to adequately spread out the remaining part of the lung. All these features of polysegmental resections increases the risk of intraoperative and postoperative complications. Also the presence of two or more wound surfaces in the lung after polysegmental resection is a causative factor of prolonged air leak. Therefore, aerostasis should be done carefully. To achieve a good aerostasis effect special membranes, surgical glue, and staplers with buttress material can be used.

It should be noted that in this group of operations most often it is necessary to use various methods of reducing the volume of hemithorax for prevention of the delayed lung expansion and residual pleural cavity, as well as the prevention of exacerbation of TB in the operated lung, is the next characterological feature of combined anatomic lung resections. The authors recommend implementation of the intraoperative pneumoperitoneum, that is, insufflation of air into the abdominal cavity through the diaphragm in a volume up to 1500 cm^3 with a specialized needle with a valve as an additional element of the operation. Recently, the authors are rarely use phrenic nerve clamping, which causes an irreversible paresis of the diaphragmatic nerve and a more severe decrease in the functional reserves of the lung (today there is no clear evidence of the usefulness of this method and the authors do not recommend it for widespread use).

The authors often apply intrapleural or postoperative corrective upper-posterior thoracoplasty, mostly in cases of dissemination of the lung. Technically, the operation is performed without additional access with subperiosteal isolation of the posterior segments of the upper 3 or 4 ribs, with the preservation of the intercostal muscles. Extapleural thoracoplasty in the postoperative period is performed during the first postoperative month from the posterior access with additional myoplasty, which maximizes the cosmetic effect of such operations.

During the 5 years of follow-up, a persistent recovery was observed in 70.2% of patients, which is a good indicator, taking into account the initial prevalence of the TB process as well as the high incidence of drug-resistant MTB in this group of patients.

Pneumonectomy

Among lung resections for TB, pneumonectomy and pleuropneumonectomy constitute up to 12% to 15%. Pneumonectomy is indicated in patients with totally destroyed lung by TB and secondary irreversible lesion localized in the most segments of the affected lung. Taking into consideration the complexity and high level of postoperative complications, particularly life-threatening complications after pneumonectomy in TB patients with extensive severe fibrous lesion of the lungs, this operation has to be considered a high-risk procedure. During 2015 to 2016, 39 adults with unilateral cavitary pulmonary TB underwent pneumonectomy. Indications for pneumonectomy only were established in all cases by a multidisciplinary team; 21 patients had positive sputum smears on MTB before surgery. Operating time varied from 95 minutes to 360 minutes. Overall operating time was associated with the prevalence and density of pleural adhesions. Blood loss varied from 50 mL to 500 mL. The intraoperative complications rate was 5.13%. Sometimes operative blood loss may be significant due to damage to the pulmonary or chest wall vessels. In authors series of pneumonectomies, this was in two cases: damage of intercostal arteries and the azygos vein (blood loss was 2-3.5 liters). The complications rate according to The Ottawa Thoracic Morbidity & Mortality System Classifying Thoracic Surgical Complications was 30.8%. Sputum smear conversion in the early postoperative period was achieved in all cases. Only the drug resistance (MDR and XDR) notably mattered ($P<0.5$). According to the authors' experience, pneumonectomy is an effective and safe procedure in complex treatment of cavitary pulmonary TB with acceptable morbidity and absence of mortality. MDR and XDR are significant risk factors for developing complications.[10]

FEATURES OF MINIMALLY INVASIVE SURGERY

Global trends in thoracic surgery are associated primarily with a decrease in operating injury and an increase in rehabilitation after surgical interventions. Nevertheless, minimally invasive operations for pulmonary TB are rarely used. Several investigators explain this fact by the long-term specific inflammation caused by MTB. Irreversible lesions, as a result of chronic process, are associated with a high risk of conversions and morbidity in the perioperative period.

The authors' group was the first who investigated and published the robotic approach for pulmonary resections in TB patients. Elective indications for robotic surgery were the same as for VATS.[7]

The results of the comparative study VATS versus robot-assisted thoracic surgery (RATS) lobectomy were published for the first time in

2018; 104 patients were included in the study and 95% of lobectomies were completed with mini-invasive access. There was no intraoperative and postoperative mortality. The frequency of conversions was the same in both groups and did not depend on the choice of access and technique of operation. The frequency of access conversion in robot-assisted lobectomies was comparable with VATS and significantly less than in published studies of mini-invasive lobectomy in pulmonary TB. At the same time, conversions were performed more often in patients with chronic obstructive pulmonary disease, which is probably due to worse technical conditions for performing lobectomy on the background of insufficient collapse of the operated lung.[1,4,11]

Multivariate analysis revealed a significant effect of the severity of chronic obstructive pulmonary disease on the conversion to a thoracotomy. In this study, the shorter duration of the surgery corresponded to a significantly lower incidence of postoperative atelectasis of the part of the lung after robotic-assisted operations, which may be explained by a negative effect of single pulmonary ventilation. The use of the robotic surgical system provided a reliable reduction in the duration of the overall operative time and the volume of intraoperative blood loss. The postoperative surgical complication rate was the same in both groups (13% and 14% for VATS and RATS respectively).

The results of the 5-year experience showed the efficacy and safety of minimally invasive lobectomies. The choice of robot-assisted operations is accompanied by a significant decrease in the frequency of pulmonary complications as well as a shorter overall operation time and less blood loss compared with VATS lobectomy.[11]

PITFALLS OF ROBOTIC ACCESS FOR PULMONARY TUBERCULOSIS

Pitfalls of robotic surgery include features of the robotic surgical system and features of pulmonary TB. Working on a Da Vinci Si surgical system (PS3000, Intui-tive Surgical) is associated with simple movements in the apex of pleural cavity and difficult working in the supradiaphragmatic area. At the same time, the possibility of division of adhesions in all parts of pleural cavity is a necessary condition for successful surgery in TB cases, which is associated with a high rate of adhesions. The authors made a choice between completely portal robotic lobectomy technique and VATS-based approach in favor of the latter. Initially the scheme proposed by Dylewski and colleagues was used.[12] The modification of this scheme consisted in maximally close position of the thoracic ports to the diaphragm, which provided freedom of movement in all parts of the pleural cavity and, especially important, provided adequate visualization and separation of pulmonary-diaphragmatic adhesions.

Another feature of the technique was the method of installing an additional (assistant) port in such a way as to prevent conflicts of assistant and robotic tools as much as possible (according to the triangle rule). In addition, the elasticity of 9 to 10 intercostal spaces, together with the lack of a developed muscular framework in this area, allowed the specimen to be removed without an extended intersection of the

Table 1
Early outcomes of surgical treatment of pulmonary tuberculosis

Authors and Year	Number of Patients	Morbidity/Mortality, %	Success Rate, %
Orki et al,[14] 2009	55	29/1.8	95
Park et al,[15] 2009	19	NA/0	79
Yu et al,[16] 2009	133	17.3/2.3	90.2
Kang et al,[17] 2010	72	15/1.4	90
Bouchikh et al,[22] 2013	29	10/0	88.23
Vashakidze et al,[18] 2013	75	9/5.5	90 (XDR) 67 (MDR)
Xie et al,[19] 2013	43	23.3/0	93
Wang et al,[20] 2017	54	11/0	87
Yablonskiy et al,[10] 2017	39 (pneumonectomy)	30.8/0	100
Kudriashov et al,[11] 2018	104 (lobectomy)	VATS 13/0 RATS 14/0	100

intercostal muscles. The preference of the anterior or posterior approach to the hilum can also influence to the choice of surgical approach and the port placement. Traditional Russian school of thoracic surgery is associated with anterior approach. Potentially, the authors have used this access in majority of cases.

Five years after begining of the robotic program for pulmonary TB, authors mark three basic techniques for division of pleural adhesions: completely robotic (if adhesions is local), standard VATS (good technique for begining surgery in cases of total obliteration of pleural cavity) and robotic redocking procedure. Last technique for effective division of pleural adhesions under the diaphragm was described in 2017. In standard cases robotic cart approaches patient from the left/right side of the head at a 15° angle. The target point for surgical system localized in the apex of pleural cavity in this position. To move the target point above the diaphragm, the authors placed the patient cart from the left/right side of the head at a 175-185 angle Camera and assistant ports remained in their places. Left and right instrumental ports were changed between themselves. Robot-assisted thoracoscopic division of adhesions over the diaphragm was more comfortable in this position of the patient cart. After pneumolysis, the patient cart was moved to the original position. This procedure increased the console operative time not more than 20 minutes.[7]

The last pitfall of robotic surgery for TB is the same as for any other pathology. Many surgeons are consider difficulties in performing conversion to a thoracotomy and slowness of the robotic system. The authors first experience of conversion access during robotic surgery was associated with large blood loss (approximately 1 L), with a background of absence of an adequate hemostasis during the performance of the thoracotomy. Subsequently, the authors started using special endoscopic sponges that allowed performing qualitative provisory hemostasis with robotic tools in cases of vascular structures injuries. This made the performance of thoracotomy more comfortable and safer compared with VATS.

POSTOPERATIVE CARE

Short-term and long-term results after surgery largely depend on careful management of patients with pulmonary TB after surgery that has already begun in the ICU. Postoperative chemotherapy is mandatory. It is important to continue the anti-TB chemotherapy after the removal of the main lung lesion, because some foci may persist and can favor relapses. The postoperative duration of anti-TB therapy is recommended by the WHO. Correction of chemotherapy is carried out according to the results of the bacteriologic study of the specimen.

The duration of postoperative chemotherapy also depends, however, on the individual clinical condition of each patient.

RESULTS OF SURGICAL RESECTION FOR PULMONARY TUBERCULOSIS

The rate of treatment success after radical resection surgery for single-sided TB ranges between 79% and 100%. The main articles during the past 10 years on this topic are presented in **Table 1**.

Immediate results of surgery for TB showed the efficacy and safety of the surgical approach. Most articles showed severity of drug resistance of MTB as a key risk factor of postoperative complications and overall success rate of the treatment.[10,11] The main benefit of TB management which includes surgical strategy is in the early conversion of excretion of MTB. This is one of the important points for improvement of the epidemiologic situation.

Scientific Evidence Proving the Correct Choice of Pulmonary Resection for Tuberculosis

A cohort retrospective-prospective study was performed by Taras Voronchihin at the St. Petersburg State Research Institute of Phthisiopulmonology between 2005 and 2012; 194 patients with fibrous-cavernous pulmonary TB were included.[13] There were 3 groups:

1. Patients who underwent a conservative strategy
2. Patients who received complex treatment with lung resection after an intensive phase of antituberculous therapy
3. Patients who received complex treatment using extrapleural thoracoplasty after an intensive phase of anti-TB therapy

The outcomes of treatment and survival, depending on the ratio of the treatment approach, were recorded and compared. The results of the study showed that the surgical method on the background of the adequate anti-TB chemotherapy could significantly improve the results of the fibrocavernous pulmonary TB treatment. In this trial, the clinical cure for patients after lung resection was 2 times faster than after collapse surgery (thoracoplasty).

Results for Surgery in Cases of Bilateral Pulmonary Tuberculosis

Surgical treatment of bilateral TB is not unusual today. Certainly, palliative surgery can alleviate the suffering of these patients, with a 40% to 60% successful rate. In several well-selected cases, however, surgery in combination with adequate antituberculous therapy can lead to a cure. In this group, as with unilateral TB, it is preferable to use minimally invasive access for earlier rehabilitation of the patient.[7]

Many patients with bilateral cavitary TB were treated in the chest center of St. Petersburg State Research Institute of Phthisiopulmonology. The value and limits of surgery in patients with advanced TB were investigated carefully. A retrospective study of 57 consecutive patients who underwent thoracic surgery for culture-positive bilateral cavitary pulmonary TB was performed. Forty-four (77.2%) patients were men and 13 (22.8%) patients were women; their ages were in the range of 18 years to 61 years. Twenty-two (38.6%) patients had MDR-TB and 35 (61.4%) patients had XDR-TB confirmed with cultures. On admission, 49 (86.0%) patients had sputum smear microscopy positive for acid-fast bacilli. The main indication for surgery was treatment failure manifested as contagious persisting cavities despite the best available therapy. The surgical procedures included combinations of pulmonary resections of different levels, selective thoracoplasty, and/or endobronchial valve treatment. The operations were performed consecutively, starting with the most affected side. TB therapy preceded the operation for a minimum of 6 months and was continued after the operation on the basis of a patient's susceptibility to drugs for MTB. The authors performed 121 operations: 42 in 22 patients with MDR-TB (1.9 operations per patient) and 79 procedures in 35 patients with XDR-TB (2.3 operations per patient). No deaths occurred in the first year. Two late deaths followed, 1 unrelated to and 1 due to TB progression. Ten major complications (1 complication per patient) developed: main bronchus stump fistula (n = 4), prolonged air leak (n = 3), respiratory failure (n = 2), and wound seroma (n = 1). At the 1-month follow-up visit, sputum smear conversion was observed in 11 (68.8%) patients with MDR-TB and in 15 (45.5%) patients with XDR TB. At the late (20–36 months) follow-up visit, culture negativity was achieved in 21 (95.5%) patients with MDR-TB and in 23 (65.7%) patients with XDR-TB ($P = .015$).

The trial showed that thoracic surgery may significantly improve patients' outcomes and even result in a cure in a good portion of patients with bilateral cavitary MDR-TB and XDR-TB and should be considered the essential element of multimodality treatment of MDR-TB and XDR-TB, even in patients with bilateral cavitary disease and borderline respiratory reserves.[21]

UNSOLVED PROBLEMS OF LUNG RESECTION FOR PULMONARY TUBERCULOSIS

The authors hope that the data given in this article will make the indications for lung resection more clear. Nevertheless, one of the issues that requires further evidence is surgery for TB without cavity and without excretion of MTB (residual lesion or sequelae of TB).

At the moment, surgery for TB without cavity is not proved and can be considered only as a possible option in treatment. The most indication is persistent radiological lesion (tuberculomas) after an adequate course of anti-TB treatment. Timing for surgery is the same as for cavitary TB. The main purpose of surgical treatment is elimination of the source of MTB to prevent possible relapses.[4] Another indication for surgery is described in the authors' previous publication as a chance to identify real drug resistance in a patient who never had excretion of MTB.[11]

According to the literature, tuberculomas sized between 1 cm and 10 cm are estimated as among the most frequent benign nodules, representing up to 25% of all resected single pulmonary nodules. In resected tuberculoma, MTB strains can be isolated in approximately 85% of cases. They may include a cavity or calcifications, and margins are usually smooth and sharp. Because of increased glucose metabolism caused by granulomatous inflammation, they can accumulate fludeoxyglucose F 18 during PET; then, they could be misdiagnosed with pulmonary tumors. The level of standardized uptake value can help carefully select patients for pulmonary resection and patients for medication treatment only.[3]

RECOMMENDATIONS FOR FUTURE RESEARCH

The WHO consensus document on TB surgery was published in 2014.[1] Nevertheless the majority of the problems of TB surgery remained the same as they were. The main research directions that would help solve the problems of TB surgery are as follows:

- Randomized trial of treatment patients with residual TB lesion (with tuberculoma and

cavities without any excretion of MTB), who will be treated by anti-TB chemotherapy alone and in combination with surgery
- Studies that will help obtain evidence of the influence of an adjusted anti-TB treatment course (based on drug susceptibility testing of MTB from the surgical specimen) on the outcomes of postoperative treatment
- Development of a single terminology source (glossary) for TB surgery

SUMMARY

Surgery successfully complements and improves the results of therapeutic treatment of pulmonary tuberculosis, especially in cases of MDR- and XDR-tuberculosis. When choosing the type of operation, it is necessary to consider the factors: the duration of the disease, the form of pulmonary tuberculosis, the number of affected lungs (single-sided or bilateral tuberculosis), functional reserves and comorbidities. Minimally invasive approaches are preferred and show good results in comparison to traditional thoracotomy. Further studies should clarify some particular issues, but the overall role of resection surgery is indisputable.

REFERENCES

1. World Health Organization. The role of surgery in the treatment of pulmonary TB and multidrug- and extensively drug-resistant TB. Geneva (Switzerland): WHO; 2014. p. 1–23.
2. World Health Organization. Global tuberculosis report 2018. Geneva (Switzerland): WHO; 2018. p. 1–147.
3. Subotic D, Yablonskiy P, Sulis G, et al. Surgery and pleuro-pulmonary tuberculosis: a scientific literature review. J Thorac Dis 2016;8(7):E474–85.
4. Yablonskii PK. Primeneniye khirurgicheskikh metodov v lechenii tuberkuleza legikh. Torakal'naya khirurgiya: natsional'nyye klinicheskiye rekomendatsii. [[Use of surgical methods in treatment of a pulmonary tuberculosis. Thoracic surgery: national surgical references]]. Moscow: GEOTAR-Media; 2014. p. 1–160 [in Russian].
5. Halezeroğlu S, Okur E. Thoracic surgery for haemoptysis in the context of tuberculosis: what is the best management approach? J Thorac Dis 2014; 6(3):182.
6. Yen YT, Wu MH, Cheng L, et al. Image characteristics as predictors for thoracoscopic anatomic lung resection in patients with pulmonary tuberculosis. Ann Thorac Surg 2011;92(1): 290–5.
7. Yablonskii P, Kudriashov G, Vasilev I, et al. Robot-assisted surgery in complex treatment of the pulmonary tuberculosis. J Vis Surg 2017;3(18):1–8.
8. Repin Ju M. Lekarstvenno-ustojchivyj tuberkulez legkih. [[Drug-resistant pulmonary tuberculosis]]. Saint-Petersburg (Russia): Gippokrat; 2007. p. 1–168 [in Russian].
9. Savin IB, Bel'tjukov MV. Prognosticheskoe znachenie perfuzionnoj scintigrafii legkih v hirurgicheskom lechenii tuberuleza. [[Prognostic value of perfusion scintigraphy in surgical treatment of pulmonary tuberculosis]]. Luchevaja Diagnostika Terapija 2017;3:84–5 [in Russian].
10. Yablonskiy P, Vasilev I, Kirjuhina L, et al. Immediate results of pneumonectomies in patients with unilateral localization of destructive pulmonary tuberculosis. Results of the prospective, non-randomized study. Medicinskij Alliance 2017;4:103–11 [in Russian].
11. Kudriashov GG, Vasilev IV, Ushkov AD, et al. Immediate results of minimally invasive lobectomy for localized single-sided pulmonary tuberculosis: comparison of robot-assisted and video-assisted approaches. Medicinskij Alliance 2018;1:51–9 [in Russian].
12. Dylewski MR, Ohaeto AC, Pereira JF. Pulmonary resection using a total endoscopic robotic video-assisted approach. Semin Thorac Cardiovasc Surg 2011;23(1):36–42. WB Saunders.
13. Voronchihin T, Avetisyan A, Vasil'ev I, et al. Results of complex treatment of limited fibrous-cavernous pulmonary tuberculosis. Medicinskij Alliance 2018;3: 56–64 [in Russian].
14. Orki A, Kosar A, Demirhan R, et al. The value of surgical resection in patients with multidrug resistant tuberculosis. Thorac Cardiovasc Surg 2009;57(04): 222–5.
15. Park SK, Kim JH, Kang H, et al. Pulmonary resection combined with isoniazid-and rifampin-based drug therapy for patients with multidrug-resistant and extensively drug-resistant tuberculosis. Int J Infect Dis 2009;13(2):170–5.
16. Yu DP, Fu Y. Surgical treatment of 133 cases of multidrug-resistant pulmonary tuberculosis. Zhonghua Jie He He Hu Xi Za Zhi 2009;32(6):450–3.
17. Kang MW, Kim HK, Choi YS, et al. Surgical treatment for multidrug-resistant and extensive drug-resistant tuberculosis. Ann Thorac Surg 2010;89(5): 1597–602.
18. Vashakidze S, Gogishvili S, Nikolaishvili K, et al. Favorable outcomes for multidrug and extensively drug resistant tuberculosis patients undergoing surgery. Ann Thorac Surg 2013;95(6): 1892–8.
19. Xie B, Yang Y, He W, et al. Pulmonary resection in the treatment of 43 patients with well-localized, cavitary pulmonary multidrug-resistant tuberculosis in

Shanghai. Interact Cardiovasc Thorac Surg 2013; 17(3):455–9.

20. Wang L, Xia F, Li F, et al. Pulmonary resection in the treatment of multidrug-resistant tuberculosis: a case series. Medicine 2017;96(50):e9109.

21. Marfina GY, Vladimirov KB, Avetisian AO, et al. Bilateral cavitary multidrug-or extensively drug-resistant tuberculosis: role of surgery. Eur J Cardiothoracic Surg 2018;3:618–24.

22. Bouchikh M, Achir A, Caidi M, et al. Role of pulmonary resections in management of multidrug-resistant tuberculosis. A monocentric series of 29 patients. Rev Pneumol Clin 2013;69(6): 326–30.

Modern Collapse Therapy for Pulmonary Tuberculosis

Denis V. Krasnov, MD, PhD[a,b,*], Sergey V. Skluev, PhD[c,d],
Yana K. Petrova, PhD[a], Dmitry A. Skvortsov, PhD[a],
Vladimir A. Krasnov, MD, PhD[b,e], Irina G. Felker, PhD[c],
Nikolay Grischenko, MD, PhD[a]

KEYWORDS

- Collapse therapy • Pulmonary tuberculosis • TB-HIV coinfection • Endobronchial valve
- Thoracoplasty

KEY POINTS

- Endobronchial valve (EbV) installation leads to faster bacteriologic conversion and cavity closure in multidrug-resistant (MDR)–tuberculosis (TB) patients; it significantly improves the efficacy of complex antituberculosis treatment. EbV application also made it possible to improve the effectiveness of the complex treatment in TB–human immunodeficiency virus patients.
- A new modification of osteoplastic thoracoplasty performed with a minimally invasive approach has been proposed to be used in the treatment of destructive tuberculosis.
- Osteoplastic thoracoplasty performed with a minimally invasive approach supplemented by EbV application is allowing the increase of effectiveness of complex anti-TB therapy, even in very complicated cases.

INTRODUCTION

Tuberculosis (TB), particularly multidrug-resistant (MDR) TB and TB–human immunodeficiency virus (HIV) coinfection, remains a major public health concern worldwide. Although the European Region of World Health Organization (WHO) accounts for less than 5% of TB cases worldwide, about 25% of the worldwide burden of MDR TB occurs in this region. Of the 30 countries classified as having a high burden of MDR TB, 9 are in the European Region of WHO. Extensively drug-

Disclosure Statement for Conflicts of Interest: Authors of this publication certify that no party having a direct interest in the results of the research supporting this article has or will confer a benefit on us or on any organization with which we are associated. Authors of this publication certify that all financial and material support for this research and work are clearly identified in the title page of the article. One of the studies reported in this publication (Endobronchial valve application in patients with TB-HIV coinfection) was supported by the grant of the President of the Russian Federation MD-7123.2015.7.

[a] Surgical Department, Federal State Budgetary Institution, Novosibirsk Tuberculosis Research Institute, Ministry of Health of the Russian Federation, Okhotskaya Street 81a, Novosibirsk 630040, Russian Federation; [b] Tuberculosis Department, Novosibirsk State Medical University, Faculty of Professional Development and Professional Retraining of Doctors, Krasnyi Prospect 52, Novosibirsk 630091, Russian Federation; [c] Endoscopy Department, Federal State Budgetary Institution, Novosibirsk Tuberculosis Research Institute, Ministry of Health of the Russian Federation, Okhotskaya Street 81a, Novosibirsk 630040, Russian Federation; [d] Treatment Faculty, Tuberculosis Department, Novosibirsk State Medical University, Krasnyi Prospect 52, Novosibirsk 630091, Russian Federation; [e] Director of the Federal State Budgetary Institution, Novosibirsk Tuberculosis Research Institute, Ministry of Health of the Russian Federation, Okhotskaya Street 81a, Novosibirsk 630040, Russian Federation
* Corresponding author.
E-mail address: krasnov77@bk.ru

Thorac Surg Clin 29 (2019) 47–58
https://doi.org/10.1016/j.thorsurg.2018.09.005
1547-4127/19/© 2018 Elsevier Inc. All rights reserved.

resistant (XDR) TB is estimated to occur in 23.4% of all MDR TB cases subjected to second-line drug-susceptibility testing. At the same time, in 2016, according to the WHO report, 476,774 cases of TB in HIV-positive patients were registered all around the world.[1] Against the background of HIV infection, *Mycobacterium tuberculosis* drug resistance is registered with a higher frequency, reaching an extremely high level (from 38.5% to 76.1%–82.1%).[2]

All mentioned conditions: MDR TB or XDR TB, TB-HIV, and MDR TB-HIV or XDR TB-HIV coinfection, call for a special approach to the anti-TB chemotherapy, as well as to the antiretroviral chemotherapy (ARVT). The treatment of these patients is rather difficult because the patient needs to take a large number of medicines (4–6 anti-TB and 3–4 antiretroviral drugs), between which there are some drug interactions.[3] In addition, low adherence to the therapy, difficulties with the availability of effective second-line anti-TB drugs in some settings, and specific features of the TB process on the late stages of HIV-infection with a severe immunodeficiency cause low effectiveness of anti-TB chemotherapy.[4–6] Mostly such patients cannot be successfully cured by conventional chemotherapy only; they need a modern approach with the use of minimally invasive therapeutic and surgical techniques directed at smear negativity.

This article discusses modern collapse therapy for patients with pulmonary TB (MDR TB and XDR TB) and TB-HIV coinfection. It describes the results of 3 independent clinical studies that prove the increased effectiveness of anti-TB chemotherapy with the use of 2 modern techniques: endobronchial valve (EbV) (MedLung, Barnaul, Russian Federation) application and osteoplastic thoracoplasty (OT) with a minimally invasive approach.

Statistical analysis in all 3 clinical trials was carried out using Statistica 10.0 (Dell Software, Austin, TX, USA) and Statistical Package for the Social Sciences 18.0 software (IBM Corp, Armonk, NY, USA). The authors calculated the average, standard deviation, or standard error. Under normal distribution (the Kolmogorov-Smirnov test), the statistical significance of differences (P values) was determined using the Pearson's χ^2 test, the Mann-Whitney U test, and the Wilcoxon paired test. If entered into a 2 by 2 table, the Fisher's exact test (FT) and the 2-tailed Fisher (TTF) exact test were used to obtain P values. Differences were considered statistically significant at $P<.05$. To determine the chances of a favorable outcome, the odds ratio (OR) and 95% confidence interval (CI) were calculated.

ENDOBRONCHIAL VALVE IN THE TREATMENT OF PULMONARY DESTRUCTIVE MULTIDRUG-RESISTANT–TUBERCULOSIS

Data regarding the EbV application in treating various pulmonary diseases have recently been published in the medical literature. This drug-free minimally invasive method is used to reduce lung volume in patients with pulmonary emphysema,[7] to treat pneumothorax in patients with bronchopleural fistulas and/or in postoperative patients,[8,9] and to treat spontaneous pneumothorax of different causes. In Russia, EbV has been used to treat patients with various forms of destructive pulmonary TB for more than 15 years.[10–12] This method was recognized as the safe and effective technique.[13,14] EbV application is actively used in more than 240 TB clinics and hospitals in Russia and some post-Soviet Union countries (http://medlung.ru/).

The objective of the present study is to study the effect of EbV as an intervention among patients with destructive pulmonary MDR TB.

Endobronchial Valve Installation Technique

The EbV is a hollow cylinder made from medically inert rubber composite material (**Fig. 1**). The valve's inner bore is round and has a smooth surface, with a nylon strut at 1 side and a falling petal valve on the other, and it is lockable owing to significant external pressure and its own elastic properties. Two-thirds of the valve's outer surface consists of thin plate radial petals, securing the device within the bronchus.

The choice of valve size depends on the diameter of the draining bronchus where it is to be placed (ie, main, lobar, segmental, subsegmental); it should exceed the diameter of the bronchus by 1.2-fold to 1.5-fold. The requisite EbV size is determined after visual assessment of the bronchial tree by comparing its diameter with that of the bronchoscope. We also use endobronchial forceps of different types and sizes to assess bronchus diameter, measuring the distance between the fully open jaws. The valve allows for unidirectional outflow of air and sputum during expiration and coughing.

Procedure of endobronchial valve installation

EbV installation is carried out under local anesthesia combined with medical sedation of the patient in the presence of an anesthesiologist. The average procedure lasts approximately 35 minutes (**Figs. 2** and **3**).

After valve installation, the endoscope is introduced into the bronchial tree in the appropriate area. The valve was then fixed by using biopsy

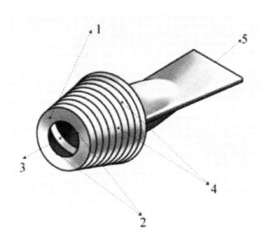

Fig. 1. EbV structure. (1) The hollow cylinder. (2) Valve inner bore. (3) Strut for grasping. (4) Radial petals for fixing the valve in the bronchus. (5) Falling petal valve. (MedLung, Barnaul, Russian Federation).

forceps (bronchoscopy) on the strut and secured to the lumen of the bronchus with visual confirmation. The radial plate petals of the valve model allow for tight fixation of the valve in the bronchial lumen. While holding the valve in the bronchus, the bronchoscope is then withdrawn from the valve (**Fig. 4**).

Effectiveness of Endobronchial Valve Installation in Multidrug-Resistant–Tuberculosis Patients

Materials and methods

The authors conducted an open comparative interventional randomized clinical trial to evaluate the efficacy of the EbV to treat MDR TB. The study was conducted in the Novosibirsk Tuberculosis Research Institute (Novosibirsk, Russian Federation) from January 2008 to December 2014. Subjects with similar clinical, laboratory, and radiological results were randomized into 2 study groups using Statistica 6.0. All subjects had documented destructive MDR TB and had received appropriate second-line anti-TB treatment in accordance with their drug-resistance pattern for more than 12 months before being enrolled into the study; this included subjects with treatment failure. All subjects were smear-positive and had not demonstrated bacteriologic conversion for the previous 6 months. Chemotherapy for all subjects included a combination of at least 5 first-line or second-line anti-TB drugs according to the individual drug-resistance patterns. Chemotherapy regimens between the 2 groups were comparable.

A total of 102 subjects were included in the study. Sample size was determined based on the results of previous studies,[10] study power (β-10%), and the high risk of loss to follow-up (low treatment adherence). The intervention group included 49 destructive MDR TB subjects who received an EbV in addition to the complex second-line treatment. The control group included 53 subjects who were administered appropriate conservative complex anti-TB treatment without EbV. The primary endpoint of the study was bacteriologic conversion and cavity closure within 365 days after EbV installation. The primary safety endpoint consisted in reducing the number of complications observed in subjects within 365 days of the procedure. EbV (certified in the Russian Federation and Europe) was installed in the appropriate lobe bronchus corresponding to the primary cavitation and to the related destructive pathologic condition. Indication for EbV installation was progressive destructive MDR TB with no bacteriologic conversion in the previous 6 months. Indications for EbV withdrawal were stable bacteriologic conversion (≥3 months), complications caused by EbV, absence of any effect of EbV for 3 months, or preparation for surgical treatment.

For subjects in both groups, evaluation of treatment efficacy was conducted synchronously, in

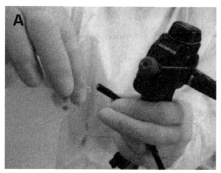
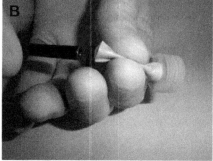

Fig. 2. Method of valve installation via endoscope (MedLung, Barnaul, Russian Federation). (*A*,*B*) Installation of EbV on the bronchoscope.

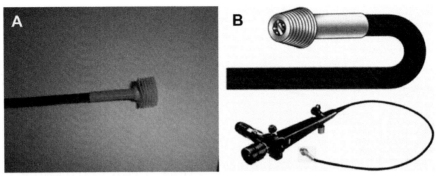

Fig. 3. Bronchoscope with the EbV (MedLung, Barnaul, Russian Federation).

accordance with the order of the Russian Ministry of Health (order #951 dated 29 December 2014) and WHO recommendations.[15] A cured case was defined as a subject who had completed treatment with no evidence of failure and 3 or more consecutive negative cultures taken at least 30 days apart after the intensive phase of treatment. Long-term results were evaluated 3 years after EbV removal in the intervention group, or 3 years after the subject's discharge from hospital in the control group. Long-term treatment results were evaluated based on criteria for clinical cure, progression of TB disease or death.

Results

The proportion of male subjects was 36.3%. This was not due to deliberate selection but because of the overall trend in hospital admissions, which was reflected in the randomized distribution. The largest age group was 21 to 30 years (n = 76, 74.5%). The average age of subjects enrolled in the study was 29.8 plus or minus 11.0 years (age 18–64 years). Rare cough, which resolved without further intervention, was observed in 12 subjects in the intervention group (24.5%). Four (8.2%) subjects experienced dry cough, dyspnea on exertion and intermittent elevations of temperature (up to subfebrile readings). These subjects required additional symptomatic drug therapy. Exacerbation of chronic obstructive pulmonary disease (COPD) requiring bronchodilator therapy occurred in 4 (8.2%) subjects. All of these symptoms resolved within 3 weeks after EbV installation. No complications occurred during the procedure. In the time immediately following EbV fixation (2 hours), the valve migrated into the lower divisions of the bronchial tree in 3 subjects. This complication was believed to have been due to an incorrect assessment of the diameter of the bronchus. This complication was remedied using a repeat procedure with the correct valve size.

During application of the EbV, special attention was paid to the speed of bacteriologic conversion and the effect of EbV on radiographic changes. It is important to highlight the high percentage of subjects with bacteriologic conversion in the intervention group: 47 (95.9%) within the first 3 months of study enrollment compared with only 20 (37.7%) subjects in the control group (P<.0001).

Serial control radiograph examination revealed that most, 27 (55.1%), subjects had hypoventilation in the blocked area, whereas 13 (26.5%) had complete atelectasis. However, hypoventilation was not observed after EbV placement in 9 (18.4%) subjects. Despite the absence of any signs of hypoventilation, 2 subjects had cavity closure. EbV was ineffective in 7 subjects; in 5 of these an increase in cavity size was observed without growth of the infiltrative component. TB progression was observed in 1 subject, and 1 person had no dynamic changes. Cavity closures were recorded in 33 (67.3%) cases in the intervention group and in 11 (20.7%) cases in the control group (relative risk [RR] 2.72, 95% CI 2.3–3.14) (**Fig. 5**).

The duration of EbV occlusion in the intervention group was 201.6 plus or minus 14.77 days. Cavity closures within the first 3 months of treatment occurred in most, 27 (55.1%), subjects in the intervention group versus only 2 (3.8%) subjects in the control group (P<.0001). Cavity closures in the intervention group occurred within 113.7 plus or minus 23.5 days versus 134.4 plus or minus 13.0 days in the control group (P = .003). The speed of cavity closure did not correlate with cavity size: in the intervention group the Spearman correlation coefficient was 0.154 (P = .3) versus 0.07 in the control group (P = .68).

In subjects with halted TB progression, reduction in cavity size, and partial infiltrate resorption following EbV intervention, the condition of 3 (37.5%) subjects stabilized and a positive trend was noted, whereas 5 (62.5%) had severe

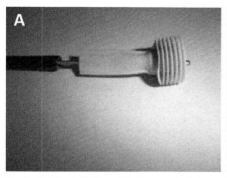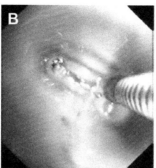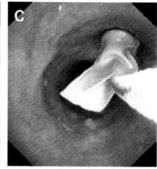

Fig. 4. EbV installation. (*A*) Removal of the valve from the bronchoscope by forceps. (*B*) Valve removal from the distal endoscope (endophoto). (*C*) Endoscope withdrawal from bronchial valve (endophoto) (MedLung, Barnaul, Russian Federation).

pulmonary fibrotic changes, with fibrous strands extending to the pleura and cavities developing in the fibrous walls. These subjects were prepared for surgery and partial lung resection was performed (see **Fig. 5**). Residual changes in a blocked bronchus were assessed after EbV removal. Immediately after EbV removal, proliferation of granulation at the site of the contact between the valve body and the bronchial wall was observed in all 49 subjects.

Long-Term Results

Long-term improvement in treatment results occurred in 77 (75.5%) subjects: 41 (83.7%) in the intervention group and 36 (67.9%) in the control group. The follow-up period lasted 3 years. A total of 42 (54.5%) MDR TB subjects from both groups were cured: 33 (80.5%) in the intervention group and 9 (25.0%) in the control group (RR 3.44, 95% CI 2.79–4.08). Relapse was observed in 5 (6.5%) subjects: 2 (4.9%) in the intervention group and 3 (8.3%) in the control group ($P = .43$). We also analyzed subjects with TB progression during long-term (3-year) follow-up. TB progression was observed in 30 (38.9%) subjects: 6 (14.6%) in the intervention group and 24 (66.7%) in the control group (RR 3.72, 95% CI 3.01–4.43).

This study shows that EbV intervention in patients with pulmonary TB is safe and potentially reversible, and is associated with a low complication rate; no intervention-associated mortality was observed in this study. The use of this procedure contributes to stabilization and improvement of the TB process. In conclusion, EbV interventions can lead to reversible changes in respiratory function, and complications are rare and reversible. EbV installation leads to faster bacteriologic conversion and cavity closure in MDR TB patients. Therefore, it may be assumed that it significantly improves the efficacy of anti-TB treatment.

ENDOBRONCHIAL VALVE IN THE COMPLEX TREATMENT OF PATIENTS WITH TUBERCULOSIS AND HUMAN IMMUNODEFICIENCY VIRUS COINFECTION

It is well known that TB-HIV coinfection is characterized by the low efficacy of anti-TB therapy and a high number of adverse treatment outcomes (37%–50%), including rare closure of the cavities (less than in 40% of patients with destructive TB processes). This situation requires research into new methods to increase the effectiveness of comprehensive TB-HIV therapy.

The purpose of the presented clinical trial was to study the possibility of increasing the efficacy of anti-TB therapy in TB-HIV patients by EbV application.

Materials and Methods

The authors conducted an open comparative interventional randomized clinical trial. The study was conducted in the Novosibirsk Tuberculosis Research Institute (Novosibirsk, Russian Federation) from January 2013 to January 2017. After consultation with a thoracic surgeon, subjects with similar clinical, laboratory, and radiological results were randomized into 2 study groups.

A total of 125 TB-HV subjects were enrolled in the study, subjects were randomly divided into 2 groups. The main group (n = 68) included subjects with destructive pulmonary TB-HIV coinfection who received an EbV in addition to the complex anti-TB therapy. The control group included 57 subjects with destructive pulmonary TB-HIV coinfection who were administered appropriate conservative complex anti-TB treatment without EbV. The effectiveness of the complex therapy was assessed in the main group after EbV removal. In the control group it was assessed after 12 to 15 months from the moment of inclusion in

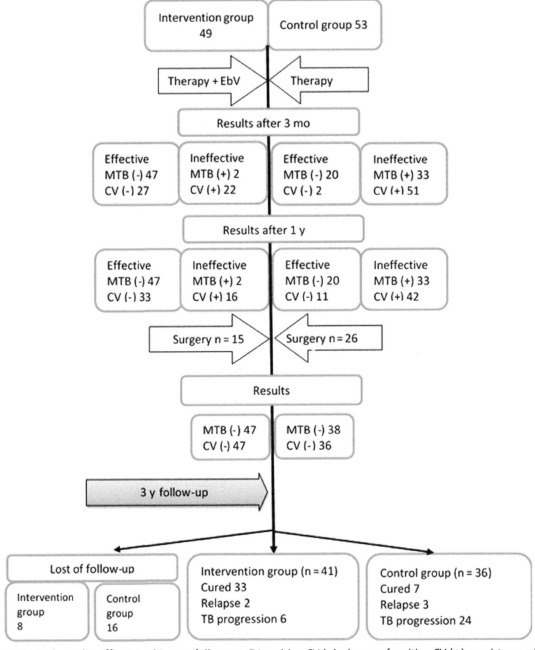

Fig. 5. Study results: efficacy and 3 years follow-up. CV, cavities; CV (−), closure of cavities; CV (+), persistence of cavities; MTB, *M tuberculosis*; MTB (−), bacteriologic conversion; MTB (+), biological specimen is positive by smear microscopy culture.

the study. We used the following assessment methodology based on clinical, radiological, and laboratory tests: considerable improvement, improvement without dynamics, deterioration, and death.

Considerable improvement was defined as bacteriologic conversion and closure of the cavities. The category of improvement included subjects who had decreases in the cavities size, bacteriologic conversion, or demonstrated significant decrease in the number of *M tuberculosis* in a sputum. The category without dynamics was defined as a lack of clinical, radiological or laboratory dynamics despite the treatment. The category of deterioration was defined as clinical and radiological progression of TB process despite of ongoing therapy.

Results

Subjects of both groups were comparable by sex, age, and social characteristics. Most of them were young men (79.4% vs 82.4, P = 0.67, χ^2) from 20 to 40 years old (76.4% vs 68.4%, P = 0.31, χ^2) who were urban dwellers (72% vs 87.7%, P = 0.03, χ^2). Nearly half of all subjects were previously in prison: 36 (52.9%) of the main group and 30 (44.1%) of the control group (P = 0.97, χ^2). The average duration of the pulmonary TB in both groups was 12 to 18 months (P = .32, the Mann-Whitney U-test).

All subjects in the both groups had destructive forms of pulmonary TB and were smear-positive by microscopy and/or culture despite the ongoing complex adequate chemotherapy. Most subjects had drug-resistant strains of M tuberculosis, 45 (69.2%) and 31 (59.6%) of cases had MDR TB strains (P = 0.28, χ^2).

The registered average duration of HIV infection was 28 months (from 22 to 40 months) in the main group and 26 months (from 20 to 43 months) in the control group (P>.05, Mann-Whitney U-test). To determine the stage of HIV infection, the viral load and the level of CD3, CD4, and CD8 lymphocytes were assessed, then the level of immunosuppression was estimated by the number of CD4+ cells in both groups. All examined subjects had IVB stage of HIV infection. ARVT was prescribed to 43 subjects of the main group and to 41 subjects of the control group. Unfortunately, due to the low adherence, only 26 (60.4%) subjects of the main group and 24 (58.5%) subjects of the control group received ARVT (P = .66, χ^2).

All main group subjects received complex adequate anti-TB chemotherapy with EbV application. During the EbV installation, no complications were registered. During the first day after the manipulations, 1 subject experienced a migration of the valve to the lower divisions of the bronchial tree. Endoscopic removal of the migrated valve and reinstallation was performed. The complication did not recur.

Based on radiograph results, 1 to 3 days after the EbV application, 82.3% of cases registered hypoventilation in the blocked zone. The average duration of EbV occlusion in the main group was 488 days and ranged from 10 to 19 months. The timing of temporary EbV occlusion in each subject was determined individually, taking into account the spread of the TB process, clinical and radiological dynamics, and speed of bacteriologic conversion. The effectiveness of treatment was assessed in the main group after EbV removal and in the control group after 12 months from the moment of inclusion in the study.

EbV application in addition to the complex anti-TB therapy achieved bacteriologic conversion in 51 (75%) of TB-HIV main group subjects. At the same time, complex adequate anti-TB chemotherapy led to bacteriologic conversion in only 24 (42%) of control group subjects (OR = 4.13, 95% CI 3.50–4.75, P = 0.0002, χ^2).

Depending on the degree of immunosuppression (number of CD4+ cells), the frequency of bacteriologic conversion was different. Among the subjects with the number of CD4+ cells less than 100 cells/μL, bacteriologic conversion was registered in 5 main group subjects (50.0% of subgroup with the number of the CD4+ cells <100 cells/μL) and in 3 (33.3%) control group subjects (P = 0.65, TTF). Among the subjects with the number of CD4+ cells from 100 to 350 cells/μL, bacteriologic conversion was achieved in 37 (74.0%) main group subjects and in 12 (33.3%) control group subjects (P = 0.0001, χ^2). Among the subjects with the number of CD4+ cells more than 350 cells/μL, all main group subjects (n = 8) and 9 (75%) of the control group subjects had bacteriologic conversion (P = 0.24, TTF).

Regardless of the degree of immunosuppression, closure of cavities in the main group with EbV was registered more frequently than in the control group: 38 (55.9%) versus 16 (28.1%), respectively (OR = 3.25, 95% CI 1.53–6.87, P = 0.0004, χ^2).

The frequency of cavities closure was different depending on the degree of immunosuppression. Among the subjects with the number of CD4+ cells less than 100 cells/μL, closure of cavities was registered in 1 main group subject (10,0% of subgroup with the number of the CD4+ cells <100 cells/μL) and in 2 (22.2%) control group subjects (P = 0.58, TTF). Among the subjects with the number of CD4+ cells from 100 to 350 cells/μL, closure of cavities was achieved in 29 (58.0%) main group subjects and in 5 (13.9%) control group subjects (P = 0.00004, TTF). Among the subjects with the number of CD4+ cells more than 350 cells/μL, all main group subjects (n = 8) and 9 (75%) of the control group subjects achieved closure of cavities (P = 0.24, TTF).

Thus, the EbV application has made it possible to improve the effectiveness of the complex treatment in TB-HIV subjects (**Table 1**). All deaths were due to the HIV infection.

OSTEOPLASTIC THORACOPLASTY WITH A MINIMALLY INVASIVE APPROACH

The main operations in TB surgery are lung resections designed to remove the main lesion foci.[15,16] However, because of various factors, lung resection may not be performed for all TB patients; it

Table 1
Results of complex antituberculous therapy in tuberculous and human immunodeficiency virus patients

	Groups				
	Main Group		Control Group		
Result	Abs.	%	Abs.	%	P
Considerable improvement	38	55.9	16	28.1	.0004[a]
Improvement	13	19.1	8	14.0	.48[b]
Without dynamics	9	13.2	20	35.1	.005[b]
Deterioration	7	10.3	11	19.3	.20[b]
Death	1	1.4	2	3.5	.59[b]
Total	68	100	57	100	—

[a] χ^2 Pearson's test.
[b] Fisher's exact test.
Abbreviation: Abs, absolute number.

is contraindicated for many. Collapse thoracoplasty may be performed on patients with contraindications to a lung resection.[15] Thoracoplasty has been performed to treat pulmonary TB for more than 100 years and had been successfully used all over the world before invention of the first anti-TB drugs.[17] Using this method has again become a necessity in the countries with a high burden of MDR TB and XDR TB. However, the collapse surgical operations developed and described over the preceding decades are accompanied by a large number of complications: an expressed pain syndrome, a significant cosmetic defect, and a resulting low adherence of patients to this method of treatment.

Therefore, at the Novosibirsk Tuberculosis Research Institute, more than 7 years ago, a group of investigators developed and are successfully using a new sparing method of OT with a minimally invasive approach that is different from the conventional method in its low degree of invasion, the absence of a cosmetic defect, less intraoperative blood loss, and fewer postoperative complications. The topographic-anatomic justification of a minimally invasive approach for OT, as well as detailed description the of surgical technique, indications, and contraindications for OT, were given in the previous publications.[18] To increase the collapse and effectiveness of OT, the authors proposed the additional EbV application in a postoperative period.

Materials and Methods

A prospective cohort trial was held in the thoracic clinic of the Novosibirsk Tuberculosis Research Institute. The trial started in January 2007 and ended in December 2013. The results assessed in the clinical trial included the clinical and laboratory parameters comparing subjects undergoing minimally invasive OT (MIOT) with conventional OT (COT).

The following criteria were applied: smear negativity and closure of the cavities in the lungs. The volume of intraoperative blood loss was assessed, as well as the postoperative complications that occurred. Direct results of the surgical treatment were evaluated with the subjects under study 12 and 18 months after the OT, based on the clinical data, radiograph images, and laboratory tests. The following categories of the results were chosen: considerable improvement, improvement, deterioration of the condition, and death.

Considerable improvement was defined as elimination of cavities and bacteriologic conversion. The category of improvement included subjects in whom the general condition normalized, the sepsis resolved, the smear became negative or the amount of purulent sputum decreased, the dissemination and perifocal inflammatory foci fully or partly resolved, and the size of the cavities decreased. The category of deterioration was defined as postoperative clinical progression of the TB infection.

Long-term results 2 to 4 years after OT were analyzed. The intermediate-term results of surgical treatment were evaluated from the clinical cure criteria of formation of a chronic TB process, progress of TB, and death.

Results

In total, 414 subjects with destructive pulmonary TB were involved in the trial. The main group consisted of 191 subjects. Of these, 105 were diagnosed with pulmonary TB more than 2 years before enrollment in the trial and 86 were diagnosed less than 2 years before enrollment. The control group consisted of 223 subjects.

By the time of admission to the surgical department, all the subjects had destructive TB, with bilateral cavities in 43 (22.5% ± 3.0%) subjects of the main group and 61 subjects (27.4% ± 3.0%) of the control group ($P = .26$, χ^2). Radiological signs of continuous progression of pericavitary infiltrates with extensive dissemination of bacteria in the lung segments were presented in most subjects: in 167 (87.4% ± 2.4%) main group subjects and in 179 (80.3% ± 2.7%) control group subjects. The TB process in the other subjects was described as unstable with frequent exacerbations in 24 (12.6% ± 2.4%) main group and 44 (19.7% ± 2.7%) control group subjects ($P = .05$,

χ^2). Cavities were most often found in the upper lobe or in the upper lobe and the superior segment of the lower lobes. Cavities in the lower lobe of those subjects in whom upper lobectomies were previously performed were found in 13 (6.8% $\pm$ 1.8%) main group and 19 (8.5% $\pm$ 1.9%) control group subjects ($P = .52$, χ^2). Multiple cavernous lesions of the lung tissue (2 or more cavities) were found in 118 (61.8% $\pm$ 3.5%) subjects of the main group and 138 (61.9% $\pm$ 3.3%) subjects of the control group ($P = .98$, χ^2). Bilateral subtotal dissemination of bacteria in the lungs was found in 178 (93.2% $\pm$ 1.8%) and 213 (95.5% $\pm$ 1.4%) cases, respectively ($P = .30$, χ^2). New infiltrates were found in the opposite lung in 39 (20.4% $\pm$ 2.9%) main group and 42 (18.8% $\pm$ 2.6%) control group subjects ($P = .69$, χ^2).

Despite the specific intense chemotherapy, nearly all subjects were smear-positive before the operation: 179 (93.7% $\pm$ 1.8%) main group and 207 (92.8% $\pm$ 1.7%) control group subjects ($P = .72$, χ^2). Among the subjects with drug resistance of the pathogen, MDR was registered in 136 (88.9% $\pm$ 2.5%) main group and in 161 (86.1% $\pm$ 2.5%) control group subjects ($P = .44$, χ^2). In more than half of the subjects with drug resistance, XDR TB was observed in 99 (64.7% $\pm$ 3.9%) main group and 106 (56.7% $\pm$ 3.6%) control group subjects ($P = .13$, χ^2).

Because of the abundance of the process in the lungs and the commonly occurring concomitant COPD, manifestations of respiratory insufficiency were observed in a significant number of the subjects in both groups. The main parameters of respiratory function complied with the normal values only in 44 (23.1% $\pm$ 3.1%) and 45 (20.2% $\pm$ 2.7%) subjects, respectively ($P = .48$, χ^2). Concomitant COPD was found in 32 (16.8% $\pm$ 2.7%) cases in the main group and in 51 (22.9% $\pm$ 2.8%) cases in the control group ($P = .12$, χ^2).

Impairment of the tracheobronchial tree is an important factor in the severity of the condition of the observed subjects. Purulent endobronchitis was diagnosed in 142 (74.3% $\pm$ 3.2%) main group cases and in 159 (71.3% $\pm$ 3.0%) controls, rendering the surgical method difficult and essentially prolonging the duration of the preoperative preparation period ($P = .49$, χ^2). Specific TB impairment of the tracheobronchial tree was found in 112 (58.6% $\pm$ 3.6%) main group cases and in 110 (49.3% $\pm$ 3.4%) controls ($P = .06$, χ^2).

Thus, the most difficult subjects with destructive pulmonary TB, those with an unstable and wave-like TB process with frequent exacerbations causing continuous progress of the disease, were included in the study.

No notable preoperative differences were found among subjects from both groups. Persistent sepsis, intense bacterial excretion, specific TB impairment of the tracheobronchial tree, and signs of respiratory insufficiency determined inadequacy of the specific chemotherapy administered to the subjects and accounted for contraindications to resection surgery. Under the existing conditions, the osteoplastic collapse thoracoplasty proved to be the operation of choice selected among the available surgical assistance methods.

A total of 196 MIOTs were performed on the subjects of the main group, whereas 238 COTs were performed on the subjects of the control group. Bilateral surgical operations were performed on 5 (2.6% $\pm$ 1.2%) subjects of the main group and on 15 (6.7% $\pm$ 1.7%) subjects of the control group ($P = .05$, χ^2). In both groups, the 5-rib variant of the operation prevailed: in 159 (81.1% $\pm$ 2.8%) and 205 (86.1% $\pm$ 2.2%) cases ($P = .16$, χ^2).

Complications and Concerns

MIOT reduced intraoperative blood loss to 400 mL in 187 (95.4% $\pm$ 1.5%) subjects in the main group. In subjects operated with the conventional approach, intraoperative blood loss of less than 400 mL occurred in 105 (44.1% $\pm$ 3.2%) cases (RR 10.10, 95% CI 9.20–11.01, $P = .0001$, χ^2). Significant intraoperative blood loss (>500 mL) occurred in 1 (0.5% $\pm$ 0.5%) case of the main group and in 69 (29.0% $\pm$ 2.9%) subjects of the control group ($P = .0001$, χ^2). Mean intraoperative blood loss during OT was 278 plus or minus 20 mL in the main group and 438 plus or minus 22 mL among controls ($P<.05$).

Traumatic pneumothorax was the only intraoperative complication occurring in 10 (5.1% $\pm$ 1.6%) main group and 28 (11.8% $\pm$ 2.1%) control cases ($P = .05$, χ^2). Traumatic pneumothorax was eliminated by drainage, ensuring a favorable outcome of the operation, so the operative plan was not changed. The postoperative course was complicated in 28 (14.7% $\pm$ 2.6%) main group subjects and in 69 (30.9% $\pm$ 3.1%) control group subjects ($P = .0001$, χ^2). The risk of complications in the early postoperative period in doing COT was higher (RR 1.46, 95% CI 1.38–1.54). Severe complications, such as hemorrhage into the extrapleural space, an extensive postoperative wound infection, progression of TB followed by respiratory insufficiency, and hypostatic pneumonia, occurred in 14 (7.3% $\pm$ 1.9%) main group subjects and 49 (22.0% $\pm$ 2.9%) controls ($P = .0001$, χ^2).

An extensive wound infection originating from the extrapleural zone took place in 3 (1.6% ± 0.9%) main group and 5 (2.2% ± 1.0%) control group subjects ($P = .45$, FT). These wounds were managed with irrigation and removal of the fragments of resected ribs. The outcome of these complications was positive.

In 1 (0.5% ± 0.5%) main group and 10 (4.5% ± 1.4%) control group cases ($P = .01$, FT), postoperative drainage revealed hemorrhage in the extrapleural space: operative exploration by thoracotomy was performed in all subjects. In all cases, diffuse bleeding was found from the cavity walls, whereas there was no hemorrhage from the large vessels. In most subjects, hemorrhage was stopped by using modern hemostatic approaches and means. In 2 control cases, continuing hemorrhage required local application of swabs and irrigation with 5% solution of the έ-aminocaproic acid. The swabs were removed on the second or third day. The hemorrhage did not recur.

In 8 (4.2% ± 1.5%) main group and 12 (5.4% ± 1.5%) control group cases, we registered postoperative pneumonia in the operated lung ($P = .37$, FT). The use of inhalation therapy, wide-spectrum antibiotics, and postural drainage enabled successful treatment of the complications in all cases.

Progressive pulmonary TB accompanied by respiratory insufficiency occurred after OT in 6 (3.1% ± 1.3%) cases of the main group and 22 (9.9% ± 2.0%) control cases ($P = .005$, FT). Correction of the anti-TB therapy ensured stabilization of the process in 2 main group cases and in 11 control group cases. Thus, statistically relevant differences were found between the groups for the rate of postoperative hemorrhage ($P = .01$, FT) and TB progression ($P = .005$, FT).

Furthermore, to increase the effectiveness of collapse therapy, the EbV was installed after thoracoplasty in most subjects of both groups: 163 (85.3% ± 2.6%) and 191 (85.7% ± 2.4%), respectively ($P = .93$, χ^2). There were few complications after this procedure, and they were removed easily.

Outcomes

The early outcome was evaluated 12 and 18 months after the OT, and the intermediate-term outcome after 2 to 4 years.

The use of MIOT was associated with bacteriologic conversion in 144 (80.4% ± 2.9%) subjects during the next 12 months after the surgery. Among subjects with COT, bacteriologic conversion was recorded for 124 (69.3% ± 3.5%) subjects (OR 1.84, 95% CI 1.72–1.97, $P = .01$, χ^2).

During the first year after thoracoplasty, closure of the cavities was observed in 159 (83.2% ± 2.7%) cases with MIOT; it was frequently at a higher rate than in the control group, with 156 cases (70.0% ± 3.0%; OR 2.13, 95% CI 1.98–2.28, $P = .002$, χ^2).

At 18 months after surgery, 173 (90.6% ± 2.1%) main group subjects were reported to have considerable improvement of their condition, whereas 14 (7.3% ± 1.9%) main group cases had an improved condition. In the control group, these figures are statistically notably lower: considerable improvement was observed in 176 (78.9% ± 2.8%) subjects ($P = .001$, χ^2) and improvement was recorded in 35 (15.8% ± 2.4%) subjects ($P = .009$, χ^2) (**Table 2**).

Clinical cure in subjects who underwent OT was observed in the intermediate term in 169 (88.5% ± 2.3%) cases and in 179 (79.7% ± 2.7%) controls ($P = .016$, χ^2) (**Table 3**).

Table 2
Results of treatment 18 months after the surgery

	Groups					
	Main Group		Control Group			
Result	Abs.	%	Abs.	%		P
Considerable improvement	173	90.6 ± 2.1	176	78.9 ± 2.8		.001[a]
Improvement	14	7.3 ± 1.9	35	15.8 ± 2.4		.009[a]
Deterioration	4	2.1 ± 1.0	11	4.9 ± 1.5		.2[b]
Death	0	0	1	0.4 ± 0.3		—
Total	191	100	223	100		—

[a] χ^2 Pearson's test.
[b] Fisher's exact test.

Table 3
Results of treatment of 2 to 4 years after osteoplastic thoracoplasty

| | Groups | | | | |
| | Main Group | | Control Group | | |
Result	Abs.	%	Abs.	%	P
Clinical cure	169	88.5 ± 2.3	177	79.7 ± 2.7	.016[a]
Formation of a chronic process	15	7.9 ± 2.0	30	13.5 ± 2.3	.066[a]
Progress of TB	6	3.1 ± 1.0	13	5.9 ± 1.6	.14[b]
Death	1	0.5 ± 0.5	2	0.9 ± 0.6	.56[b]
Total	191	100	223	100	—

[a] χ^2 Pearson's test.
[b] Fisher's exact test.

Thus, comprehensive treatment that included surgical collapse therapy with MIOT increased the chances of achieving clinical cure (OR 1.09, 95% CI 1.05–1.12), compared with the conventional surgery. The authors emphasize that these intermediate term results occurred in a difficult category of subjects who had severe clinical manifestations of the disease and unstable courses of the TB process, who had low adherence to chemotherapy, and who presented a high epidemiologic hazard for the community.

SUMMARY

The treatment of MDR TB, XDR TB, and TB-HIV combination patients presents many challenges, including both patients' motivation to adhere to and comply with treatment protocols and the problem of tolerability of anti-TB drugs and ARVT. The novel approaches and sparing techniques, such as EbV application and performing the MIOT developed by the authors, allowed us to increase the effectiveness of complex anti-TB therapy. In a century when existing anti-TB drugs are not as effective as before, we have to use all possibilities to fight TB. Achieving the required selective concentric collapse of the lung tissue in patients with destructive pulmonary TB and especially in patients with drug resistance or/and with HIV coinfection leads to the bacteriologic conversion; cavity closure; and, in the end, to the successful cure.

ACKNOWLEDGEMENT

The study reported in this publication (Endobronchial valve application in patients with TB-HIV coinfection) was supported by the grant of the President of the Russian Federation MD-7123.2015.7.

REFERENCES

1. WHO. Global tuberculosis report 2017 – URL. Available at: http://www.who.int/tb/publications/global_report/en/. Accessed April 02, 2018.
2. Khazova E.Yu., Ivanova NA Complexities of diagnosis and treatment of patients with HIV-associated tuberculosis. Bulletin of medical Internet conferences 2014;4(5):813. [in Russian].
3. Federal clinical guidelines for the diagnosis and treatment of tuberculosis in patients with HIV infection. Moscow (Russia); 2014. p. 28. [in Russian]. Available at: file:///D:/Downloads/Federalnye-klini-cheskie-rekomendatsii.pdf. Accessed March 29, 2018.
4. Zimina VN, Vasilieva IA, Batyrov FA, et al. The effectiveness of chemotherapy in patients with tuberculosis and HIV co-infection. Tuberculosis and Lung Diseases 2013;3:15–21 [in Russian].
5. Mordyk AV, Ivanova OG, Sitnikiva SV, et al. Tuberculosis in combination with HIV infection: the reasons for failures in treatment. Omsk Scientific Bulletin 2015;2(144):23–6 [in Russian].
6. Dobkina MN, Solovyova SA, Chernov AS, et al. The treatment of patients with HIV/TB co-infection in Tomsk region. Tuberculosis and Lung Deseases 2014;1:91 [in Russian].
7. Shah PL, Slebos DJ, Cardoso PF, et al. EASE trial study group. Bronchoscopic lung-volume reduction with Exhale airway stents for emphysema (EASE trial): randomised, sham-controlled, multicentre trial. Lancet 2011;378:997–1005.
8. Schweigert M, Kraus D, Ficker JH, et al. Closure of persisting air leaks in patients with severe pleural empyema - use of endoscopic one-way endobronchial valve. Eur J Cardiothorac Surg 2011;39: 401–3.
9. Giddings O, Kuhn J, Akulian J. Endobronchial valve placement for the treatment of bronchopleural

fistula: a review of the current literature. Curr Opin Pulm Med 2014;20:347–51.

10. Krasnov DV, Grishchenko NG, Beschetnyy TG, et al. The use of valve stem bronchus blockade in patients with advanced fibro-cavernous pulmonary tuberculosis after osteoplastic thoracoplasty. Tuberc Lung Dis 2010;9:8–13 [Russian].

11. National Association of TB Specialists, Association of Thoracic Surgery of Russia. National clinical guidelines on the use of surgical techniques in the treatment of pulmonary tuberculosis. Moscow (Russia): Russian Federation: Association of Thoracic Surgery of Russia; 2013 [in Russian].

12. Levin AV, Tseymakh EA, Nikolaeva OB, et al. Collapsotherapeutic methods in the complex treatment of patients with destructive infiltrative pulmonary tuberculosis with drug resistance of the pathogen. Tuberculosis Lung Dis 2013;12:65–9 [in Russian].

13. Popova LA, Shergina EA, Lovacheva OV, et al. Functional response to the endobronchial valve installation in patients with destructive pulmonary tuberculosis. Tuberculosis Lung Dis 2016;94(9):30–8 [in Russian].

14. Sklyuev SV, Krasnov DV. Evaluation of the influence of endobronchial valve installation on the respiratory function on the example of patients with infiltrative destructive pulmonary tuberculosis. Pulmonology 2013;5:49–52 [in Russian].

15. World Health Organization. The role of surgery in the treatment of pulmonary TB and multidrug and extensively drug resistant TB. Geneva (Switzerland): WHO; 2014.

16. Yablonsky PK, Sokolovich EG, Avetisyan AO, et al. The role of thoracic surgery in the treatment of pulmonary tuberculosis (literature review and the authors' observations). Med Alliance J 2014;3:4–10 [in Russian].

17. Barker WL. Thoracoplasty. Chest Surg Clin N Am 1994;4(3):593–615.

18. Krasnov D, Krasnov V, Skvortsov D, et al. Thoracoplasty for tuberculosis in the twenty-first century. Thorac Surg Clin 2017;27(2):99–111.

Nontuberculous Mycobacteria
Epidemiology and the Impact on Pulmonary and Cardiac Disease

Wendi K. Drummond, DO, MPH,
Shannon H. Kasperbauer, MD*

KEYWORDS

- Nontuberculous mycobacteria • Epidemiology • Pulmonary disease • Endocarditis
- Heater-cooler unit

KEY POINTS

- Nontuberculous mycobacteria are ubiquitous in the environment, making surveillance difficult.
- The most common nontuberculous mycobacterial species include slow growing mycobacteria such as *Mycobacterium avium* complex and *Mycobacterium kansasii*, followed by rapidly growing mycobacteria such as *Mycobacterium abscessus* and *Mycobacterium chelonae*.
- Population-based data suggest that the prevalence is increasing in the United States and worldwide.
- Host factors are important in disease risk and include the presence of underlying structural lung disease, rheumatoid arthritis, and underlying immunodeficiency, including immunosuppressive medications.

INTRODUCTION

This article reviews the epidemiology and impact of nontuberculous mycobacteria (NTM)-related pulmonary disease (NTM-PD). Although the epidemiology of mycobacterium tuberculosis is well-described, the epidemiology of pulmonary NTM infections is less well-defined in the United states and other areas of the world. *Mycobacterium tuberculosis* is known to cause disease via person-to-person transmission. We do not have definitive evidence to support that NTM are transmitted person to person, although there is molecular evidence of emerging dominant clones of *Mycobacterium abscessus* in the cystic fibrosis population that could be transmitted via fomites or aerosols.[1]

Current studies support that disease caused by NTM are far more prevalent than formerly appreciated. Nontuberculous mycobacteria are in the same family as tuberculosis but occupy a vastly different environmental niche. Clinical manifestations are similar among the different NTM species. Because these are ubiquitous organisms in the environment, they can be difficult to study from an epidemiologic perspective. Additionally, NTM-PD is not uniformly a reportable disease; therefore, it is difficult to evaluate the scope of clinical disease in humans. It is also challenging to determine whether or not the isolation of an organism from a clinical specimen represents infection (presence of the pathogen in the airways) versus disease that causes clinical illness and morbidity.

Disclosure Statement: The authors have nothing to disclose.
Department of Medicine, National Jewish Health, 1400 Jackson Street, Denver, CO 80206, USA
* Corresponding author.
E-mail address: kasperbauers@njhealth.org

Thorac Surg Clin 29 (2019) 59–64
https://doi.org/10.1016/j.thorsurg.2018.09.006
1547-4127/19/© 2018 Elsevier Inc. All rights reserved.

NTM are ubiquitous in the environment and have been isolated from surface water, soil, tap water, domestic and wild food products, and milk.[2,3] They can thrive within municipal water systems in a biofilm, and it is suspected that NTM infect a susceptible host via inhalation of an aerosol.[4]

CLINICAL SYNDROMES

Generally speaking, NTM cause 4 distinct clinical syndromes: pulmonary disease, skin and soft tissue infections, disseminated disease, and lymphadenitis. In the United States, pulmonary disease is primarily caused by *Mycobacterium avium* complex (MAC), and *Mycobacterium abscessus* is the second most common species. Skin and soft tissue infections are usually the consequence of direct inoculation from trauma and may be associated with surgical procedures. Disseminated disease is usually seen in immune compromised patients, such as in patients with AIDS or other immune compromising conditions. Importantly, disseminated disease has been associated with the global outbreak of *Mycobacterium chimaera* infections related to heater-cooler unit contamination in operating theaters.[5] Superficial lymphadenitis is most commonly caused by MAC or *Mycobacterium scrofulaceum* in children and *M tuberculosis* in adults.[6]

PULMONARY DISEASE

There are 2 major radiographic presentations of NTM lung disease, most commonly associated with MAC:

- Fibrocavitary disease, with a pattern similar to tuberculosis which typically occurs in males with chronic obstructive pulmonary disease (COPD) related to smoking. This usually manifests as disease in the upper lobes of the lungs.
- Bronchiectatic nodular disease, which involves bronchiectasis, nodules and occurs primarily in women without underlying pulmonary disease. These women typically are nonsmokers. This is the most common presentation of MAC in the United States.

Other clinical presentations have been described including hypersensitivity pneumonitis and MAC pulmonary infections associated with solitary pulmonary nodules. Other slow-growing mycobacterial species such as *Mycobacterium xenopi*, *Mycobacterium kansasii*, *Mycobacterium szulgai*, and *Mycobacterium malmoense* present more often with cavitary lung disease.

RISK FACTORS FOR DISEASE

There are a number of risk factors for NTM pulmonary disease, with both host and environmental risk factors playing a role (**Box 1**). These pathogens are ubiquitous in the environment owing to their presence in the soil and water. Despite our frequent exposure to these environmental organisms, the disease prevalence is lower than would be expected. Therefore, host factors and host susceptibility are very important. Host factors include malignancy, underlying structural lung disease such as COPD and bronchiectasis, ciliary dysfunction, anatomic abnormalities such as thoracic skeletal issues, underlying autoimmune disease such as rheumatoid arthritis and immunosuppression associated with immunomodulatory drugs (eg, tumor necrosis factor-alpha blockers).[7,8] Environmental risk factors include exposure to regions of high water vapor content found in warm, humid environments.[9] Patients with pulmonary MAC disease have also been shown to have significantly greater soil exposure than noninfected controls.[10]

The population affected by COPD has conventionally been male and smokers, and in areas of the world where smoking is still prevalent, COPD remains an important risk factor. Individuals with cystic fibrosis are also at higher risk for NTM infection, as are individuals with bronchiectasis from other causes. The prevalence of NTM isolation in CF patients in the United States is estimated to be 13%.[11] In a study that looked at a population of Medicare beneficiaries in the United States, bronchiectasis was found to be associated with NTM pulmonary disease.[12] There was a higher prevalence of disease noted among women.

Studies have noted an association with a specific phenotype in female patients, with a tall, thin, low body mass index morphotype being predominant.[13,14] Other features of these patients with NTM lung disease were noted to have higher rates of scoliosis, pectus excavatum, and mitral valve prolapse compared with matched controls.

Host susceptibility considerations are also important in terms of risk for disease. Organ transplant recipients, patients with CD4 lymphopenia owing to human immunodeficiency virus infection or other idiopathic causes, and the use of tumor necrosis factor-alpha inhibitors are all predisposing risk factors that affect host susceptibility. Cytokines such as tumor necrosis factor-alpha are essential to granuloma formation and maintenance, and anything that interrupts this immune pathway can predispose a patient to infection.[15] Other defects in the host immune response, affecting the macrophage or T-helper type 1 cell pathway contribute to increased susceptibility to

---

Box 1
Risk factors for nontuberculous mycobacteria infection and disease

Environmental sources of mycobacteria

Soil exposure (acidic pine forest, coastal swamp soils)

Indoor swimming pool use

Hot tub use

Drainage waters from coastal swamps

Dusts from agriculture, garden and potting soils

Aerosols from indoor humidifiers

Host factors

Lung cancer or neoplasms of the trachea or bronchus

Chronic obstructive pulmonary disease

Bronchiectasis

Thoracic skeletal abnormalities

Low body weight

Rheumatoid arthritis

Immunomodulatory drugs/anti-tumor necrosis factor agents

Steroid use

Gastroesophageal reflux disease

Other immune compromising conditions (AIDS, CD4 lymphopenia, Mendelian susceptibility to mycobacterial diseases, common variable immune deficiency)

Ciliary dysfunction (primary ciliary dyskinesia)

Cystic fibrosis

Macrophage dysfunction

NTM infection. Although rare, Mendelian susceptibility to mycobacterial diseases includes a group of inherited disorders that can predispose to NTM infections. These disorders include interferon gamma receptor deficiencies, autoantibody states, and IL-12 deficiency, as examples.[16,17]

NTM clinicians appreciate an association between NTM pulmonary disease and gastroesophageal reflux. One study found that 26% of patients with the nodular bronchiectatic form of NTM-PD had gastroesophageal reflux disease based on ambulatory 24-hour esophageal pH monitoring and only 27% of these patients had typical gastroesophageal reflux disease symptoms.[18]

DISEASE FREQUENCY

The majority of species causing clinical disease in humans in the United States include members of the slowly growing mycobacteria such as MAC.

Other less common entities include *M kansasii*, *Mycobacterium marinum*, *M xenopi*, *Mycobacterium simiae*, and certain rapidly growing mycobacteria such as *M abscessus and Mycobacterium chelonae*. Estimating true disease prevalence is difficult given that the isolation of NTM from a clinical isolate does not always correlate with disease. This finding is complicated by the fact that only a few states have reporting requirements for NTM.

Because NTM are environmental pathogens that can potentially contaminate laboratory specimens, specific criteria have been established by the American Thoracic Society (ATS)/Infectious Disease Society of America (IDSA) to help determine which patients have pulmonary disease. These include clinical, radiographic, and microbiologic criteria to help distinguish clinical disease from colonization.[6]

The microbiologic diagnostic criteria include isolation of an NTM organism from 2 separate sputum cultures, or 1 bronchial lavage or a lung biopsy noting histopathologic changes consistent with mycobacterial infection and a positive NTM respiratory sample. A study by Winthrop and colleagues[19] suggested that the ATS/IDSA microbiologic criteria for NTM-PD correlated well with the ATS clinical criteria for pulmonary disease in which 86% of patients meeting the ATS/IDSA microbiologic criteria for disease also met the ATS/IDSA clinical criteria.

Disease frequency can be measured by either incidence or prevalence calculations. Incidence is the identification of new cases in a specifically defined population over a designated period of time, whereas disease prevalence is a measure of the frequency of cases in a defined population. Prevalence estimates, such a period prevalence, is a superior means by which to estimate disease burden owing to a chronic disease such as pulmonary NTM.

DISEASE TRENDS
North America

A national survey conducted from 1981 to 1983 based on isolates reported to state laboratories, estimated a disease prevalence of 1.8 per 100,000 persons. This survey noted that individuals with NTM disease were more likely to be white females over 75 years of age.[20]

NTM disease burden is increasing in the United States and other areas of the world while conversely rates of tuberculosis in developing nations are decreasing. One systematic review included 22 studies encompassing 5 different countries including the United States, Japan, Canada, Europe, Australia, and Japan over a 72-year period (1946–2014).[21] This review noted that NTM disease incidence increased in 75% of the regions examined.

Using Medicare beneficiary data from 1997 to 2007, the annual prevalence significantly increased from 20 to 47 cases per 100,000 persons, or 8.2% per year.[12] The period prevalence was 112 cases per 100,000 persons. Western states were noted to have higher rates of NTM disease, with Hawaii ranking the highest at 396 per 100,000 persons.

In a population-based study from Oregon, pulmonary disease incidence (as defined by the ATS microbiologic criteria) increased with age and increased 2.2% per year from 2007 to 2012.[22] MAC was the most common etiologic agent (88%). In those with a rapid grower, M abscessus was most frequently isolated. The mean age of study participants was 66 years old and 59% were female. Comorbid conditions included COPD, lung cancer, and bronchiectasis. NTM more frequently affected women compared with other studies, showing an increased prevalence with males associated with COPD.[23] In their study, men had more COPD or pleural effusions with the women having more immune suppression and bronchiectasis.

Examining data from 4 integrated US health systems from 2004 to 2006 revealed an NTM-PD prevalence of 1.4 to 6.6 cases per 100,000 persons, with an increase by 2.6% to 2.9% per year.[24] As in other studies, MAC was the most commonly isolated pathogen in 79% to 86% of confirmed cases, followed by M chelonae/M abscessus with a frequency of 5.2% to 19.2%. M kansasii was associated with 0.0% to 6.2% of definite cases.

Regional Differences

Europe has lower rates of NTM isolation and disease than North America. Patients in the European studies tended toward more men, younger in age. This finding is most likely thought to be related to smoking patterns with differences where in Europe, 23% of adults are smokers compared with 15% in the United States and Canada.[25]

Data collected in Africa, South American, and the Middle East have suggested that many patients thought to have chronic pulmonary tuberculosis in fact have NTM disease.[26]

Population-based data trends available from North America, Europe, New Zealand, and Australia suggest a continued increase in NTM prevalence since 2000, with North America and Australia having higher annual prevalence (3.2–9.8 per 100,000 persons) than Europe, where it is

less than 2 per 100,000.[27] Studies from East Asia including Japan, South Korea and China also show an increasing prevalence of NTM pulmonary disease.[28–30]

Global partners from NTM-Network European Trials Group (NET) provided pulmonary isolate data (2008) from 62 laboratories in 30 countries across 6 continents.[31] MAC species predominated in most countries. Important geographic differences were observed, including higher rates of rapidly growing mycobacterial recovery in Eastern Asia, whereas M xenopi was more predominant in eastern Canada and Europe.

IMPACT ON THORACIC DISEASE

Approximately 90% of NTM disease manifests as a chronic pulmonary infection. The other 10% is related to extrapulmonary infections including skin, soft tissue, lymphadenitis, and disseminated infection. The pulmonary manifestations include a chronic cough, fevers, weight loss, night sweats, dyspnea, and occasionally hemoptysis. Owing to the nonspecific and indolent nature of symptoms, some patients may be symptomatic for months or even years before they are diagnosed. Depending on the pathogenicity of the infecting strain and the host vulnerability, the clinical progression can be variable.

Strollo and colleagues[32] estimated 86,244 national cases in 2010 totaling $815 million in costs. Medical encounters among those aged 65 years and older ($562 million) were more than 2-fold higher than those younger than 65 years of age ($253 million). Using previously published growth rates of 8% per year, projected 2014 estimates resulted in 181,037 national annual cases totaling $1.7 billion in costs.

One retrospective review of 106 NTM-PD patients from the National Institutes of Health noted a mortality rate of 4.2 per 100 person-years.[33] Significant risk factors for death included fibrocavitary disease and pulmonary hypertension. Among Danish patients (mean age of 60 years), the 5-year mortality was 33.5% in NTM colonization and 40.1% in NTM disease with no statistical difference.[23]

In 2017, Marras and colleagues[34] published results from a population-based cohort study of persons with microbiologically defined NTM pulmonary disease (NTM-PD) or NTM pulmonary isolation diagnosed from 2001 to 2013 in Ontario, Canada. This study matched more than 18,000 patients who had microbiologically confirmed pulmonary NTM with unexposed controls. They demonstrated an increased risk for death in both NTM-PD and NTM pulmonary isolation. The

5-year mortality estimates were 26.6% for NTM pulmonary isolation and 36.9% for NTM-PD.

HEATER–COOLER UNIT OUTBREAK

In 2011, a case of disseminated *M chimaera* (a species of MAC) was recognized in Switzerland.[35] This patient presented with fever, weight loss, and respiratory distress 2 years after cardiac surgery. His diagnostic evaluation included negative conventional blood cultures and a normal transesophageal echocardiogram. A diagnosis of sarcoidosis was made with concomitant granulomatous hepatitis and nephritis. Unfortunately, the patient received 1 year of steroid therapy before he decompensated and was found to have disseminated mycobacterial infection related to endocarditis with positive mycobacterial cultures from multiple sites.

The source of this infection is related to contamination of the LivaNova (formerly Sorin) 3T heater cooler unit used in operating suites around the world. Other units have been found to harbor bacteria in the water reservoirs; however, it is believed that the design of the 3T heater cooler unit allows for aerosolization of the bacteria into the suite while the fans are running.[5,36]

Key clinical symptoms of this infection include fevers, malaise, weight loss, cough, and dyspnea. Common clinical signs of disseminated *M chimaera* include cytopenias, elevated inflammatory markers, transaminitis, renal insufficiency, chorioretinitis, and splenomegaly.[37] These infections often present as prosthetic valve endocarditis, but limited local infection to the sternum and soft tissues has also been reported.[37,38]

Since the recognition of the first case, more than 100 cases of heater cooler unit–related infections have been reported globally.[39] The Swiss Chimaera Taskforce estimate an annual incidence of 156 to 282 cases for the 10 major valve replacement markets and 51 to 80 cases in the United States alone.[40] The greatest challenges related to this outbreak include the prolonged latency between presentation and the prior surgery (up to 5 years postoperatively) in addition to the high mortality rate of 50%.

SUMMARY

The prevalence of this orphan disease first recognized in the 1950s is clearly growing. It is more prevalent than *M tuberculosis* in the United States and most other developed countries. NTM-PD is a chronic, progressive pulmonary infection that has an impact on morbidity and mortality. It is imperative that clinicians recognize this emerging infection.

REFERENCES

1. Bryant JM, Grogono DM, Rodriguez-Rincon D, et al. Emergence and spread of a human-transmissible multidrug-resistant nontuberculous mycobacterium. Science 2016;354(6313):751–7.
2. Goslee S, Wolinsky E. Water as a source of potentially pathogenic mycobacteria. Am Rev Respir Dis 1976;113(3):287–92.
3. Wolinsky E, Rynearson TK. Mycobacteria in soil and their relation to disease-associated strains. Am Rev Respir Dis 1968;97(6):1032–7.
4. Falkinham JO 3rd. Epidemiology of infection by nontuberculous mycobacteria. Clin Microbiol Rev 1996; 9(2):177–215.
5. Sax H, Bloemberg G, Hasse B, et al. Prolonged outbreak of mycobacterium chimaera infection after open-chest heart surgery. Clin Infect Dis 2015;61(1): 67–75.
6. Griffith DE, Aksamit T, Brown-Elliott BA, et al. An official ATS/IDSA statement: diagnosis, treatment, and prevention of nontuberculous mycobacterial diseases. Am J Respir Crit Care Med 2007;175(4): 367–416.
7. Marras TK, Daley CL. Epidemiology of human pulmonary infection with nontuberculous mycobacteria. Clin Chest Med 2002;23(3):553–67.
8. Winthrop KL, Baxter R, Liu L, et al. Mycobacterial diseases and antitumour necrosis factor therapy in USA. Ann Rheum Dis 2013;72(1):37–42.
9. Prevots DR, Adjemian J, Fernandez AG, et al. Environmental risks for nontuberculous mycobacteria. Individual exposures and climatic factors in the cystic fibrosis population. Ann Am Thorac Soc 2014;11(7):1032–8.
10. Maekawa K, Ito Y, Hirai T, et al. Environmental risk factors for pulmonary Mycobacterium avium-intracellulare complex disease. Chest 2011;140(3): 723–9.
11. Olivier KN, Weber DJ, Wallace RJ Jr, et al. Nontuberculous mycobacteria. I: multicenter prevalence study in cystic fibrosis. Am J Respir Crit Care Med 2003;167(6):828–34.
12. Adjemian J, Olivier KN, Seitz AE, et al. Prevalence of nontuberculous mycobacterial lung disease in U.S. Medicare beneficiaries. Am J Respir Crit Care Med 2012;185(8):881–6.
13. Kim RD, Greenberg DE, Ehrmantraut ME, et al. Pulmonary nontuberculous mycobacterial disease: prospective study of a distinct preexisting syndrome. Am J Respir Crit Care Med 2008;178(10):1066–74.
14. Kartalija M, Ovrutsky AR, Bryan CL, et al. Patients with nontuberculous mycobacterial lung disease exhibit unique body and immune phenotypes. Am J Respir Crit Care Med 2013;187(2):197–205.
15. Winthrop KL, Chang E, Yamashita S, et al. Nontuberculous mycobacteria infections and anti-tumor

necrosis factor-alpha therapy. Emerg Infect Dis 2009;15(10):1556–61.

16. Wu UI, Holland SM. Host susceptibility to nontuberculous mycobacterial infections. Lancet Infect Dis 2015;15(8):968–80.

17. Bustamante J, Boisson-Dupuis S, Abel L, et al. Mendelian susceptibility to mycobacterial disease: genetic, immunological, and clinical features of inborn errors of IFN-gamma immunity. Semin Immunol 2014;26(6):454–70.

18. Koh WJ, Lee JH, Kwon YS, et al. Prevalence of gastroesophageal reflux disease in patients with nontuberculous mycobacterial lung disease. Chest 2007;131(6):1825–30.

19. Winthrop KL, McNelley E, Kendall B, et al. Pulmonary nontuberculous mycobacterial disease prevalence and clinical features: an emerging public health disease. Am J Respir Crit Care Med 2010; 182(7):977–82.

20. O'Brien RJ, Geiter LJ, Snider DE Jr. The epidemiology of nontuberculous mycobacterial diseases in the United States. Results from a national survey. Am Rev Respir Dis 1987;135(5):1007–14.

21. Brode SK, Daley CL, Marras TK. The epidemiologic relationship between tuberculosis and nontuberculous mycobacterial disease: a systematic review. Int J Tuberc Lung Dis 2014;18(11):1370–7.

22. Henkle E, Hedberg K, Schafer S, et al. Population-based incidence of pulmonary nontuberculous mycobacterial disease in Oregon 2007 to 2012. Ann Am Thorac Soc 2015;12(5):642–7.

23. Andrejak C, Thomsen VO, Johansen IS, et al. Nontuberculous pulmonary mycobacteriosis in Denmark: incidence and prognostic factors. Am J Respir Crit Care Med 2010;181(5):514–21.

24. Prevots DR, Shaw PA, Strickland D, et al. Nontuberculous mycobacterial lung disease prevalence at four integrated health care delivery systems. Am J Respir Crit Care Med 2010;182(7):970–6.

25. Henry MT, Inamdar L, O'Riordain D, et al. Nontuberculous mycobacteria in non-HIV patients: epidemiology, treatment and response. Eur Respir J 2004; 23(5):741–6.

26. Maiga M, Siddiqui S, Diallo S, et al. Failure to recognize nontuberculous mycobacteria leads to misdiagnosis of chronic pulmonary tuberculosis. PLoS One 2012;7(5):e36902.

27. Prevots DR, Marras TK. Epidemiology of human pulmonary infection with nontuberculous mycobacteria: a review. Clin Chest Med 2015;36(1):13–34.

28. Ko RE, Moon SM, Ahn S, et al. Changing epidemiology of nontuberculous mycobacterial lung diseases in a tertiary referral hospital in Korea between 2001 and 2015. J Korean Med Sci 2018; 33(8):e65.

29. Morimoto K, Iwai K, Uchimura K, et al. A steady increase in nontuberculous mycobacteriosis mortality and estimated prevalence in Japan. Ann Am Thorac Soc 2014;11(1):1–8.

30. Wang HX, Yue J, Han M, et al. Nontuberculous mycobacteria: susceptibility pattern and prevalence rate in Shanghai from 2005 to 2008. Chin Med J (Engl) 2010;123(2):184–7.

31. Hoefsloot W, van Ingen J, Andrejak C, et al. The geographic diversity of nontuberculous mycobacteria isolated from pulmonary samples: an NTM-NET collaborative study. Eur Respir J 2013;42(6): 1604–13.

32. Strollo SE, Adjemian J, Adjemian MK, et al. The burden of pulmonary nontuberculous mycobacterial disease in the United States. Ann Am Thorac Soc 2015;12(10):1458–64.

33. Fleshner M, Olivier KN, Shaw PA, et al. Mortality among patients with pulmonary non-tuberculous mycobacteria disease. Int J Tuberc Lung Dis 2016; 20(5):582–7.

34. Marras TK, Campitelli MA, Lu H, et al. Pulmonary nontuberculous mycobacteria-associated deaths, Ontario, Canada, 2001-2013. Emerg Infect Dis 2017;23(3):468–76.

35. Achermann Y, Rossle M, Hoffmann M, et al. Prosthetic valve endocarditis and bloodstream infection due to Mycobacterium chimaera. J Clin Microbiol 2013;51(6):1769–73.

36. Sommerstein R, Ruegg C, Kohler P, et al. Transmission of mycobacterium chimaera from heater-cooler units during cardiac surgery despite an ultraclean air ventilation system. Emerg Infect Dis 2016;22(6): 1008–13.

37. Scriven JE, Scobie A, Verlander NQ, et al. Mycobacterium chimaera infection following cardiac surgery in the United Kingdom: clinical features and outcome of the first 30 cases. Clin Microbiol Infect 2018 [Epub ahead of print].

38. Chand M, Lamagni T, Kranzer K, et al. Insidious risk of severe mycobacterium chimaera infection in cardiac surgery patients. Clin Infect Dis 2017;64(3):335–42.

39. van Ingen J, Kohl TA, Kranzer K, et al. Global outbreak of severe Mycobacterium chimaera disease after cardiac surgery: a molecular epidemiological study. Lancet Infect Dis 2017;17(10): 1033–41.

40. Sommerstein R, Hasse B, Marschall J, et al. Global health estimate of invasive mycobacterium chimaera infections associated with heater-cooler devices in cardiac surgery. Emerg Infect Dis 2018;24(3):576–8.

Medical Management of Pulmonary Nontuberculous Mycobacterial Disease

Julie V. Philley, MD*, David E. Griffith, MD

KEYWORDS

• NTM • Nontuberculous • Mycobacteria • MAC • *Abcsessus*

KEY POINTS

- There are multiple nontuberculous mycobacterial (NTM) species isolated from respiratory specimens and many of them do not cause human disease.
- *Mycobacterium avium* complex (MAC) is the most common clinically significant NTM species isolated in the United States and can often be treated with thrice-weekly therapy.
- *Mycobacterium abscessus* is a rapidly growing mycobacterium that generally requires intravenous therapy and is difficult to eradicate.
- Clinicians must have a working knowledge of the mycobacterial laboratory to provide optimal patient management and NTM treatment regimens.

INTRODUCTION

Nontuberculous mycobacterial (NTM) pulmonary infections are commonly encountered in the United States.[1–3] The prevalence of NTM lung infection in the United States has long surpassed that of tuberculosis (TB) due to more effective antibiotic therapy for TB and initiatives, such as directly observed therapy that improved TB treatment outcomes and dramatically lowered TB incidence and prevalence. The advent and availability of CT scanning also improved NTM diagnostic capabilities and disease recognition.

There are approximately 200 identified NTM species, most of which do not cause human disease.[4] Clinicians must have sufficient familiarity with the NTM disease-causing potential of individual NTM species to accurately diagnose, treat, and follow NTM lung disease patients. Due to the rising number of diagnosed NTM cases, whether due to improved diagnostic capabilities or increased prevalence, the surgical community will undoubtedly encounter these patients more frequently. This article discusses medical management of NTM pulmonary disease patients.

DIAGNOSIS

According to the 2007 American Thoracic Society (ATS) and Infectious Diseases Society of America (IDSA) guidelines, pulmonary NTM disease is diagnosed based on a constellation of clinical symptoms, microbiologic data, and radiographic findings.[5] Symptoms may include weight loss, chronic cough, hemoptysis, night sweats, shortness of breath, and fatigue. A diagnosis requires 2 positive sputum acid-fast bacilli (AFB) cultures for the same NTM species or 1 culture-positive

Disclosure Statement: Drs J.V. Philley and D.E. Griffith have participated as on advisory boards and as consultants for Insmed pharmaceuticals.
Pulmonary and Critical Care Medicine, The University of Texas Health Science Center at Tyler, 11937 US Highway 271, Tyler, TX 75708, USA
* Corresponding author.
E-mail address: Julie.Philley@uthct.edu

Thorac Surg Clin 29 (2019) 65–76
https://doi.org/10.1016/j.thorsurg.2018.09.001

bronchial lavage specimen or tissue biopsy culture. Additionally, characteristic radiographic changes, such as nodules associated with bronchiectasis or fibrocavitary changes, must be present. If a patient does not exhibit symptoms or have characteristic radiographic changes, a sputum positive for NTM may not indicate true disease. It is necessary that clinicians understand that not all NTM respiratory isolates require antibiotic therapy nor do all patients with positive sputum cultures for NTM meet the diagnostic criteria for NTM lung disease.

TREATMENT OF NONTUBERCULOUS MYCOBACTERIAL LUNG DISEASE

Surgical intervention is unequivocally beneficial for selected patients with NTM lung disease. For all of the organisms discussed later, surgery can play an important role in patient management. In general, the more antibiotic resistant the NTM organism, the more potentially important surgical intervention may be. For multiple reasons, not least of which is adequate postoperative healing, antibiotic therapy must be optimized for every patient.

SLOWLY GROWING MYCOBACTERIA

Slowly growing mycobacteria are defined as showing evidence of growth on solid medium after more than 7 days. The slowly growing NTM species that are most commonly encountered and known to cause human disease are discussed further. Parenthetically, *Mycobacterium tuberculosis* (MTB) and *M leprae* are also slow-growing mycobacteria.

TREATMENT OF *MYCOBACTERIUM AVIUM* COMPLEX

M avium complex (MAC) is comprised of 8 species, including *M avium*, *M intracellulare*, and *M chimaera*. A majority of microbiology laboratories do not distinguish between the different MAC species because treatment regimens and clinical outcomes are similar. Some of the infrequently isolated species are not as virulent or as commonly associated with significant disease.[6]

Clinicians must be familiar with microbiologic features of MAC infections, because they differ from MTB and TB in important ways. Perhaps the most important difference, and one that is difficult for clinicians to understand, is that as opposed to MTB, the in vitro susceptibility patterns of MAC do not always correlate with or predict clinical response.[5] For this reason,

the current ATS/IDSA guidelines recommend in vitro susceptibility testing for macrolides (eg, clarithromycin and azithromycin) only as in vitro susceptibility for these drugs are the only ones that correlate with or predict treatment response. More recently, amikacin has been shown correlated with a clinical response and, therefore, may predict treatment success.[7] In contrast, in vitro susceptibilities for other drugs that are frequently used in the treatment of MAC, such as ethambutol, moxifloxacin, streptomycin, clofazimine, and the rifamycins, do not correlate with treatment response and thus their in vitro susceptibility patterns do not necessarily inform treatment management decisions. An important practical consequence of this disparity is that ethambutol is a critical element in the MAC treatment regimen regardless of the in vitro susceptibility result because it protects against the emergence of macrolide resistance. In contrast, there is no established role for moxifloxacin or other fluoroquinolones, again regardless of the in vitro susceptibility results. It is imperative that clinicians familiar with the idiosyncrasies of MAC antibiotic management be involved in their care.

There are 2 general radiographic patterns for MAC lung disease in the immunocompetent patient. The first is characterized by nodules associated with bronchiectasis, referred to as *nodular/bronchiectatic disease*. This pattern is most often seen in postmenopausal, white women with a distinct body phenotype, including mitral valve prolapse and pectus excavatum.[8–10] These patients frequently present with an insidious onset of symptoms, such as relentless cough, weight loss, fatigue, and occasional hemoptysis. Often carrying a diagnosis of chronic bronchitis or mislabeled as asthmatics, many of these individuals remain undiagnosed for many years. High-resolution CT of the chest typically reveals nodules in association with bronchiectasis, which is often primarily in the mid and lower lung zones (**Fig. 1**). Previously described as Lady Windermere syndrome, likened to Victorian women from an Oscar Wilde play, these women do not exhibit a robust cough mechanism.[11] The second typical radiographic pattern is fibrocavitary disease, which is generally upper lobe predominant (**Fig. 2**). This pattern is typically seen in patients with chronic obstructive pulmonary disease and is associated with a worse prognosis compared with the nodular bronchiectatic form of the disease.[5,12] It is important to understand the type of patient radiographic pattern of MAC lung disease to provide optimal treatment regimens.

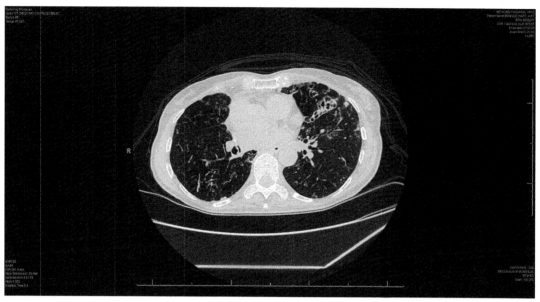

Fig. 1. Nodular bronchiectasis in a 65-year-old female patient with chronic cough.

MEDICAL THERAPY FOR NODULAR BRONCHIECTATIC *MYCOBACTERIUM AVIUM* COMPLEX LUNG DISEASE

Three-times weekly therapy with a macrolide (azithromycin, 500 mg daily, or clarithromycin, 500 mg orally, twice a day), ethambutol (25 mg/kg), and a rifamycin (rifampin, 600 mg, or rifabutin, 150–300 mg) has been shown an effective regimen in patients with nodular bronchiectatic MAC lung disease[13] (**Table 1**).

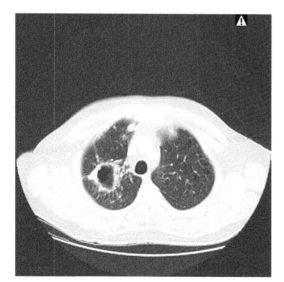

Fig. 2. Right upper lobe cavitary MAC lung disease in a patient with chronic obstructive pulmonary disease.

MEDICAL THERAPY FOR CAVITARY *MYCOBACTERIUM AVIUM* COMPLEX LUNG DISEASE

Fibrocavitary disease requires daily therapy with MAC antibiotics, including a macrolide (azithromycin, 250 mg daily, or clarithromycin, 500 mg orally, twice a day), ethambutol (15 mg/kg daily), and a rifamycin (rifampin, 600 mg, or rifabutin, 150–300 mg). The addition of a parenteral agent, such as an aminoglycoside, is also recommended, usually intravenous amikacin. The optimal dosing of the aminoglycoside is not established and should be guided by a clinician with experience managing MAC lung disease patients. Intravenous or intramuscular streptomycin is another option. Blood levels of the aminoglycoside must be followed, and side effects, such as renal toxicity, must be discussed and monitored throughout duration of use (**Table 2**).

TREATMENT OF RECALCITRANT/MACROLIDE-RESISTANT *MYCOBACTERIUM AVIUM* COMPLEX

It is critically important to prevent the emergence of macrolide resistance during MAC therapy because treatment success greatly diminishes when the MAC minimum inhibitory concentration (MIC) for macrolides is greater than 16 μg/mL.[14] Evaluation of current treatment patterns shows that many pulmonary and infectious disease specialists do not adhere to the ATS/IDSA treatment guidelines, with 1 study indicating that only 13%

Table 1
Treatment of common slowly growing mycobacteria

Nontuberculous Mycobacterial Species[a]	Drug Regimen	Duration of Therapy

MAC	Nodular/bronchiectasis:
	    Clarithromycin, 500 mg po twice daily tiw,
	        or azithromycin, 500–600 mg po tiw
	    Plus ethambutol, 25 mg/kg po tiw
	    Plus
	    Rifampin, 600 mg po daily or tiw, *or* rifabutin,
	        150–300 mg po daily or 300 mg tiw
	Cavitary: azithromycin, 250–500 mg po daily, or
	    clarithromycin, 500 mg twice daily
	    Plus
	    Ethambutol, 15 mg/kg po daily
	    Plus
	    Rifampin, 600 mg, or rifabutin, 150–300 mg po daily
	    Plus
	    An aminoglycoside: amikacin, 5–15 mg/kg IV tiw, *or*
	        streptomycin, 5–15 mg/kg IM or IV
		12 mo of negative cultures while on therapy

M kansasii	Rifampin, 600 mg po daily, *or* rifabutin, 150–300 mg po
	    daily
	    Plus
	    Ethambutol, 15 mg/kg po daily
	    Plus
	    Azithromycin, 250 mg po daily, or clarithromycin, 500 mg po
	        bid, or moxifloxacin, 400 mg po daily[b]
		12 mo of negative cultures while on therapy

M xenopi	Clarithromycin, 500 mg po bid, or azithromycin, 250 mg po
	    daily
	    Plus
	    Isoniazid, 300–600 mg po daily
	    Plus
	    Rifampin, 600 mg po daily, or rifabutin, 150–300 mg
	    Plus
	    Ethambutol, 15 mg/kg po daily
	    Plus
	    IV streptomycin or amikacin depending on
		12 mo of negative cultures while on therapy

M szulgai	Rifampin, 600 mg po daily, *or* rifabutin, 150–300 mg
	    therapy
	    Plus
	    Ethambutol, 15 mg/kg po daily
	    Plus
	    Azithromycin, 250 mg po daily, or clarithromycin, 500 mg po
	        bid, or moxifloxacin, 400 mg po daily[b]
		12 mo of negative cultures while on therapy

M simiae[c]	Sulfamethozaole (double strength) po twice daily
	    Plus
	    Amikacin, 5–15 mg/kg IV tiw
	    Plus
	    Azithromycin, 250 mg po daily, or clarithromycin, 500 mg po
	        bid or moxifloxacin, 400 mg po daily
		12 mo of negative cultures while on therapy

Abbreviations: IM, intramuscular; IV, intravenous; TIW, 3 times weekly.
[a] Peak levels should be monitored at least weekly.
[b] Isoniazid has traditionally been given in this regimen and is recommended in the 2007 ATS/IDSA guidelines but has questionable value with rifampin and ethambutol and less activity against *M kansasii* compared with newer macrolides and fluorquinolones.
[c] No therapeutic regimen of proved efficacy.

Table 2
Treatment of common rapidly growing mycobacteria

Nontuberculous Mycobacterial Species	Drug Regimen	Duration of Therapy
M abscessus subsp *abscessus*	IV amikacin, 10–15 mg/kg daily *plus* 2 of the following: IV imipenem, IV cefoxitin, IV tigecycline, Oral linezolid, 300–600 mg daily, Clofazimine, 50–100 mg daily	12 mo of negative cultures while on therapy
M abscessus subsp *massiliense*	Azithromycin, 250 mg daily *plus* IV amikacin, 10–15 mg/kg daily *plus* 1 of the following: IV imipenem, IV cefoxtin, IV tigecycline, Oral linezolid, 300–600 daily, Clofazimine, 50–100 mg daily	12 mo of negative cultures while on therapy
M abscessus subsp *boletti*	IV amikacin, 10–15 mg/kg daily *plus* 2 of the following: IV imipenem, IV cefoxtin, IV tigecycline, Oral linezolid, 300–600 daily, Clofazimine, 50–100 mg daily	12 mo of negative cultures while on therapy
M fortuitum	2 drugs based on susceptibilities Eg, sulfamethozaole, fluoroquinolones	12 mo of negative cultures while on therapy

followed current guidelines, with as many as 30% of regimens promoting macrolide resistance (eg, macrolide monotherapy, macrolide + fluoroquinolone, or macrolide + rifampin).[5,15]

Second-line agents for MAC include inhaled amikacin, clofazimine, linezolid, fluoroquinolones, and bedaquiline and are typically reserved for recalcitrant and/or macrolide-resistant disease. The role of inhaled amikacin, specifically an inhaled liposomal amikacin preparation, in a treatment regimen for advanced or recalcitrant NTM lung disease is promising.[16,17] One retrospective observational study involved administration of the inhaled generic amikacin for treatment refractory *M abscessus* and MAC patients followed for a median of 19 months[17]; 25% of these patients had sustained negative AFB cultures while receiving the inhaled generic amikacin. Patients had variable symptomatic and objective responses to the amikacin, and 35% of patients stopped amikacin due to side effects or adverse events. A multicenter, prospective, randomized clinical trial investigating the addition of inhaled liposomal amikacin to a stable regimen for recalcitrant MAC and *M abscessus* lung disease was recently completed.[18] In the study, after only

3 months of the inhaled liposomal amikacin preparation, approximately 30% of MAC patients converted sputum for AFB culture negative after a median of 1 month of therapy. The placebo-controlled and blinded phase of the study was followed by an open-label phase, which was associated with further sputum AFB culture conversion in patients who initially received placebo; 73% percent of patients had side effects or adverse events attributable to the drug and 16% discontinued the medication because of these side effects or adverse events. In this relatively small and preliminary study, it seems that the liposomal amikacin preparation has the potential to add significantly to the therapy for otherwise treatment-refractory MAC lung disease patients.

There has been little evidence to support use of fluoroquinolones in MAC lung disease. They are not considered first-line agents for treating MAC. The use of macrolide and fluoroquinolone without other companion drugs places patients at risk for development of macrolide-resistant MAC disease. Additionally, both drug classes are associated with a prolonged QT interval on an electrocardiogram, which may predispose to cardiac toxicity and excess mortality.[14,19] A recent study evaluated the effect of adding moxifloxacin in 41 MAC lung disease patients who did not have sputum conversion after at least 6 months of a macrolide-containing regimen.[20] With a median moxifloxacin administration duration of greater than 300 days, the overall treatment success rate was 29% and the median time to sputum conversion was 91 days. A positive sputum AFB smear at the start of treatment with moxifloxacin-containing regimens was an independent predictor of an unfavorable microbiologic response. This outcome has not yet been confirmed by other investigators.[21] In at least 2 studies, the addition of fluoroquinolone to the treatment regimen of macrolide-resistant MAC lung disease did not improve outcome. If fluoroquinolones had any significant activity, it would be expected to become evident in this setting.

Clofazimine, mostly used as a treatment of leprosy and multidrug-resistant TB, has gained increased use as therapy for NTM, primarily MAC and M abscessus. Limited data suggest that for patients who do not tolerate rifamycins, clofazimine may provide an effective alternative, combined with ethambutol and a macrolide.[22,23] van Ingen and colleagues[24] evaluated 564 clinical NTM isolates, including 16 clinical MAC isolates for in vitro synergy between amikacin and clofazimine. Significant synergy was demonstrated against all MAC isolates. The investigators concluded that the safety and tolerability of adding clofazimine to amikacin-containing regimens should be tested in clinical trials. Another study by Shen and colleagues[25] also reported a high synergistic effect of clofazimine used with amikacin in rapidly growing mycobacteria. Recently, 112 patients were included in a retrospective clofazimine use study.[26] A majority of the patients had MAC lung disease, including 78% who had refractory disease; 41 of 82 (50%) patients reporting treatment success defined as sputum conversion to negative cultures within 12 months but 16 patients (14%) had to stop the drug to an adverse reaction. Other studies have also found clofazimine to be effective in rapidly growing mycobacterial disease, such as M abscessus.[27] Given its high penetration in skin and soft tissue, clofazimine is often used in treatment of skin diseases and/or wound infections, many of which require surgical débridement, although data for long-term outcomes and treatment efficacy are lacking.

Bedaquiline, a Food and Drug Administration–approved drug to treat multidrug-resistant TB, has been used in MAC lung disease and seems effective for some patients and well tolerated.[28] With low MICs, further studies are warranted to understand the clinical use of bedaquiline, especially in combination with drugs such as clofazimine.[29–31]

The oxazolidinone antibiotics, such as linezolid, have been used to treat MAC lung disease without clear benefit despite in vitro activity.[32–34] Poor tolerability, including neuropathy and cytopenias, are frequently reported with linezolid.

TREATMENT OF *MYCOBACTERIUM KANSASII*

Mkansasii lung is similar in presentation to TB and is often associated with upper lobe fibrocavitary disease. Treatment outcomes with antibiotic regimens that include a rifamycin are generally good. The standard ATS/IDSA recommended therapy is a daily 3-drug regimen of isoniazid, rifampin, and ethambutol plus pyridoxine (50 mg/d). The rifampin dose is 10 mg/kg per day to a maximum of 600 mg per day, and ethambutol is given at 15 mg/kg per day. An initial 2 months of ethambutol at 25 mg/kg per day is no longer recommended. The duration of treatment is usually 18 months to 24 months, although good results with a treatment duration of 12 months whereas sputum cultures are negative have been reported. The role of isoniazid in this regimen is not clear (the MICs are 100× higher than with MTB). Clarithromycin, however, is highly active with M kansasii as it is with other slowly growing NTM species. A 3-times weekly 3-drug oral regimen (azithromycin or clarithromycin, rifampin, and ethambutol) with 12 months of culture negativity has been reported with excellent cure rates.[35] The authors favor a regimen, including rifampin, ethambutol, and macrolide. In contrast to MAC lung disease, flouorquinolones have significant in vitro and in vivo activity against M kansasii and can be used in salvage regimens for rifamycin-resistant M kansasii disease.

TREATMENT OF OTHER SLOW-GROWING NONTUBERCULOUS MYCOBACTERIAL SPECIES
Mycobacterium simiae

M simiae isolation is not always indicative of true infection.[5] The clinical presentation, including the typical accompanying symptoms, is usually similar to that of other slow-growing NTM species associated with nodular bronchiectatic disease, although cavitary disease is sometimes seen. When clinical disease is present, M simiae is difficult to treat. To date, there are no predictably effective drug combinations for treating M simiae.[36–38] A multidrug regimen based on susceptibility testing is recommended for this multidrug-resistant organism; however, many M simiae isolates show in vitro susceptibility to amikacin only or perhaps amikacin plus sulfa. Some experts recommend parenteral amikacin-based regimens with some combination of sulfa, fluoroquinolone, macrolide, and linezolid regardless of the in vitro susceptibilities. M simiae is challenging and requires expert consultation.

Mycobacterium xenopi

M xenopi lung infections are associated with high all-cause mortality with low overall survival rates.[30–39] In a retrospective study of 136 patients with M xenopi pulmonary infection from France, the absence of treatment was associated with a particularly poor prognosis; median survival was 10 months in untreated patients compared with 32 months in treated patients.[40] Combination therapy with a rifamycin-containing regimen was associated with improved survival. In a similar study from the Netherlands, multiple different treatment regimens were used in 49 patients with M xenopi lung disease, but no specific drug combination showed consistently superior results.[41] A study of M xenopi infection in nude mice found that amikacin-containing regimens were the most effective against M xenopi and that no differences were found between regimens containing clarithromycin and oxofloxacin in vivo.[42] An ethambutol/rifampin combination with clarithromycin or moxifloxacin had significant bactericidal activity against M xenopi. Although still controversial and lacking conclusive proof of superior efficacy, the current ATS/IDSA recommendation for a regimen, including rifampin/ethambutol with clarithromycin and adjunctive aminoglycoside, initially seems appropriately aggressive given the high mortality associated with M xenopi infection.[5] Although isoniazid is also recommended, it does not seem to add significantly to the other drugs in the regimen.

Mycobacterium szulgai

M szulgai is often associated with clinically significant disease in countries, such as the Netherlands, whereas fewer than half of isolates have been reported to cause significant disease in South Korea.[43,44] It is often regarded a pathogenic in the United States, especially when ATS/IDSA criteria are met. Most patients respond to a multidrug regimen, including daily azithromycin, ethambutol, and rifampin. Quinolones therapy has also been used with success in combination with ethambutol and a rifamycin.[44]

RAPIDLY GROWING MYCOBACTERIA

Rapidly growing mycobacteria are defined as organisms with observable growth on solid medium in less than 7 days. Common rapidly growing mycobacteria, which can cause lung disease, include M abscessus complex organisms, including subsp abscessus, subsp bolletii, and subsp massiliense. M chelonae is a rare cause of lung disease as is M fortuitum, noting that M fortuitum rarely causes lung disease in the absence of gastrointestinal disorders.

Mycobacterium abscessus

M abscessus is often grouped into 1 large M abscessus complex and is the most ubiquitous rapidly growing mycobacteria found in the United States.[5] The nomenclature within the M abscessus complex can be difficult to navigate, especially in light of multiple changes that have occurred.[45–49] The most recent consensus nomenclature for M abscessus complex includes M abscessus subsp abscessus, M abscessus subsp bolletii, and M abscessus subsp massiliense. This nomenclature is used for this article. M abscessus subsp abscessus is the most common rapidly growing mycobacterium isolate in North America, with 80% having an active erm 41 gene, which confers inducible macrolide resistance.[50] M abscessus subsp bolletii isolates are also macrolide resistant by this mechanism. In contrast, M abscessus subsp massiliense has an inactive erm gene and is generally macrolide susceptible as evidenced by improved clinical treatment outcomes with macrolide-containing treatment regimens.[51] Drugs that may be useful for treating M abscessus complex organisms include the macrolides (for macrolide-susceptible organisms only), linezolid, tigecycline, imipenem, amikacin, and cefoxitin.[27,32,52–58] Combination therapy is mandatory for significant disease, with the overall goal 12 months of negative sputum cultures while on therapy. For macrolide-susceptible and macrolide-susceptible M abscessus isolates, a combination of parenteral drugs should be used based on in vitro susceptibilities. Side-effect monitoring and lower doses of antibiotics are often warranted to achieve therapeutic goals (**Tables 3** and **4**).

Mycobacterium chelonae

M chelonae is a rare cause of lung disease and does not have an active erm gene, so that it is generally macrolide susceptible.

Mycobacterium fortuitum

M fortuitum is recognized as a rare cause of lung disease, almost always associated in patients with achalasia and rarely other gastroesophageal reflux disorders with recurrent aspirational lung disease.

Table 3
Common side effects of nontuberculous mycobacterial antibiotics

Nontuberculous Mycobacterial Medications	Most Common Side Effects
Macrolides (clarithromycin, azithromycin)	Nausea, vomiting, ototoxicity, QT prolongation, myopathy, granulomatous hepatitis (clarithromycin), hearing loss
Ethambutol	Visual changes/optic neuritis, peripheral neuropathy, rash, renal insufficiency
Rifamycins (rifampin, rifabutin)	Flulike illness, rash, bone marrow suppression, uveitis (rifabutin), discoloration of body fluids, hepatotoxicity, nausea, drug interactions
Aminoglycosides (streptomycin, amikacin)	Perioral numbness, eosinophilia, nephrotoxicity, ototoxicity, neurotoxicity
Clofazimine	Skin discoloration, visual changes, joint pain, eosinophilic enteritis, nausea
Fluoroquinolones	Joint or muscle pains, tendon toxicity, QT prolongation, hepatotoxicity, nephrotoxicity, rash, dizziness, headache
Bedaquiline	QT prolongation, nausea, electrolyte abnormalities
Isoniazid	Hepatotoxicity, neuropathy, jaundice, rash, neurotoxicity, optic neuritis, drug interactions, lupus-like syndrome
Tigecycline	Nausea, vomiting, diarrhea, anorexia
Cefoxitin	Rash, nausea, diarrhea
Imipenem	Nausea, rash, visual disturbances, dizziness, seizures
Linezolid	Nausea, peripheral neuropathy, myelosuppression, rash, gastrointestinal side effects, optic neuritis
Trimethoprim sulfamethoxazole	Rash, fever, myelosuppression, renal insufficiency, agranulocytosis, hepatotoxicity, myalgias
Inhaled amikacin	Tinnitus, cough, hoarseness, hearing loss

Most *M fortuitum* isolates have a functional *erm* gene, so most are macrolide resistant.[59,60] *M fortuitum* isolates are usually susceptible to fluoroquinolones, doxycycline, and minocycline (50%); sulfonamides and trimethoprim/sulfamethoxazole; and amikacin, imipenem, and tigecycline, and approximately one-half of the isolates are susceptible to cefoxitin. If the underlying gastroesophageal disorder is untreated, *M fortuitum* lung disease does not usually respond to medications.

NONPHARMACOLOGIC TREATMENT OPTIONS

Chest physiotherapy has long been used in cystic fibrosis (CF) patients to improve lung function and mucocilliary clearance.[61–64] Data for airway clearance in non-CF bronchiectasis are sparse, so recommendations are generally extrapolated from the CF literature. Airway clearance is believed effective in a majority of cases, although evidence through randomized control trials in this group are lacking.[65] Airway clearance techniques, such as use of nebulized hypertonic saline, are usually recommended recognizing there are few data showing benefit in NTM lung disease.[66,67]

In contrast to CF, recombinant human DNase has not proved effective, and evidence suggests it may possible be harmful; thus, use is not recommend.[68] Inhaled mannitol was also studied and was not proved to reduce exacerbations but seemed safe and well tolerated.[69] It was shown to increase time to exacerbations.

Mounting evidence suggests that household sources of NTM exposure, specifically household plumbing and water sources, are important for acquiring NTM pathogens.[70–74] The demonstration of likely NTM recurrence after successful NTM therapy in bronchiectasis suggests an ongoing host vulnerability and environmental exposure that seems to call for efforts to limit environmental NTM exposure.[13] It is still unknown, however, how much of a risk NTM in municipal water and household plumbing presents for the majority of patients with bronchiectasis and NTM lung disease. It is also not certain, for instance, that avoidance of aerosolized water from showers

Table 4
Dos and don'ts for nontuberculous mycobacterial lung diseases

Nontuberculous Mycobacterial Isolate	Do	Don't
MAC	• Use a multidrug regimen • Aggressively treat cavitary disease prior to surgery	• Use macrolide monotherapy • Rely on susceptibilities except for macrolides • Operate without antibiotics treatment
M kansasii	• Consider most isolates clinically significant • Use a multidrug regimen • Check rifampin susceptibilities	• Operate without antibiotic treatment
M simiae	• Obtain early expert consultation	• Assume all isolates represent true disease
M szulgai	• Consider most isolates clinically significant • Use a multidrug regimen	• Operate without antibiotic treatment
M xenopi	• Obtain susceptibilities • Aggressively treat cavitary disease	• Operate without antibiotic treatment
M abscessus	• Obtain early expert consultation • Aggressively treat disease prior to surgery • Anticipate wound healing complications	• Operate without antibiotic treatment
M fortuitum	• Consider formal gastrointestinal evaluation • Use at least 2 drugs based on susceptibilities	• Treat unless ATS guidelines are met

without avoidance of other potential aerosol-generating activities associated with running water in the home would eliminate the risk of household NTM transmission. Interventions, such as increasing the temperature of the hot water heater to greater than or equal to 130°F or changing shower heads at regular intervals might decrease risk of NTM transmission but the impact of these steps is not known.[71] It is also still unknown whether exposure to specific soil-based sources of NTM organisms may contribute to the development of NTM lung disease.[75]

Nutrition is important, especially when surgical Intervention is considered. Maintaining adequate caloric intake and body mass index and following prealbumin levels as a marker of nutrition may be helpful. Some individuals also find it helpful to take probiotic therapy while taking an antibiotic regimen for NTM disease.

Exercise, including pulmonary rehabilitation, is encouraged in individuals with chronic lung disease, including bronchiectasis.[76] Aerobic activity and deep breathing activities, such as yoga, are generally believed helpful as is pulmonary rehabilitation.

SUMMARY

Surgical intervention is often necessary for successful outcome in treatment of NTM lung disease. Successful outcomes typically involve a multidisciplinary team, including pulmonary and/or infectious disease specialist support, respiratory therapy, and nutrition support. It is also abundantly clear that for selected patients, surgical intervention improves the chances for long-term treatment success. The prevalence of NTM is rising in the United States, with newer laboratory techniques to distinguish between NTM isolates to help guide treatment regimens. Clinicians, including surgeons, are encountering NTM infections with increasing frequency and a general knowledge of common pathogens and diagnostic criteria are essential to treatment success.

REFERENCES

1. Cassidy PM, Hedberg K, Saulson A, et al. Nontuberculous mycobacterial disease prevalence and risk factors: a changing epidemiology. Clin Infect Dis 2009;49:e124–9.

2. Winthrop KL, McNelley E, Kendall B, et al. Pulmonary nontuberculous mycobacterial disease prevalence and clinical features: an emerging public health disease. Am J Respir Crit Care Med 2010; 182:977–82.

3. Prevots DR, Shaw PA, Strickland D, et al. Nontuberculous mycobacterial lung disease prevalence at four integrated health care delivery systems. Am J Respir Crit Care Med 2010;182:970–6.

4. Fedrizzi T, Meehan CJ, Grottola A, et al. Genomic characterization of Nontuberculous Mycobacteria. Sci Rep 2017;7:45258.

5. Griffith DE, Aksamit T, Brown-Elliott BA, et al. An official ATS/IDSA statement: diagnosis, treatment, and prevention of nontuberculous mycobacterial diseases. Am J Respir Crit Care Med 2007;175: 367–416.

6. Tateishi Y, Hirayama Y, Ozeki Y, et al. Virulence of Mycobacterium avium complex strains isolated from immunocompetent patients. Microb Pathog 2009;46:6–12.

7. Brown-Elliott BA, Iakhiaeva E, Griffith DE, et al. In vitro activity of amikacin against isolates of Mycobacterium avium complex with proposed MIC breakpoints and finding of a 16S rRNA gene mutation in treated isolates. J Clin Microbiol 2013;51:3389–94.

8. Kim RD, Greenberg DE, Ehrmantraut ME, et al. Pulmonary nontuberculous mycobacterial disease: prospective study of a distinct preexisting syndrome. Am J Respir Crit Care Med 2008;178:1066–74.

9. Leung JM, Fowler C, Smith C, et al. A familial syndrome of pulmonary nontuberculous mycobacteria infections. Am J Respir Crit Care Med 2013;188: 1373–6.

10. Kartalija M, Ovrutsky AR, Bryan CL, et al. Patients with nontuberculous mycobacterial lung disease exhibit unique body and immune phenotypes. Am J Respir Crit Care Med 2013;187:197–205.

11. Reich JM, Johnson RE. Mycobacterium avium complex pulmonary disease presenting as an isolated lingular or middle lobe pattern. The Lady Windermere syndrome. Chest 1992;101:1605–9.

12. Ito Y, Hirai T, Maekawa K, et al. Predictors of 5-year mortality in pulmonary Mycobacterium avium-intracellulare complex disease. Int J Tuberc Lung Dis 2012;16(3):408–14.

13. Wallace RJ Jr, Brown-Elliott BA, McNulty S, et al. Macrolide/azalide therapy for nodular/bronchiectatic mycobacterium avium complex lung disease. Chest 2014;146(2):276–82.

14. Griffith DE, Brown-Elliott BA, Langsjoen B, et al. Clinical and molecular analysis of macrolide resistance in Mycobacterium avium complex lung disease. Am J Respir Crit Care Med 2006;174:928–34.

15. Adjemian J, Prevots DR, Gallagher J, et al. Lack of adherence to evidence-based treatment guidelines for nontuberculous mycobacterial lung disease. Ann Am Thorac Soc 2014;11:9–16.

16. Davis KK, Kao PN, Jacobs SS, et al. Aerosolized amikacin for treatment of pulmonary Mycobacterium avium infections: an observational case series. BMC Pulm Med 2007;7:2.

17. Olivier KN, Shaw PA, Glaser TS, et al. Inhaled amikacin for treatment of refractory pulmonary nontuberculous mycobacterial disease. Ann Am Thorac Soc 2014;11:30–5.

18. Olivier KN, Gupta R, Daley CL, et al. A controlled study of liposomal amikacin for inhalation in patients with recalcitrant nontuberculous mycobacterial lung disease. Abstract #50985, Presented at the annual meeting of the American Thoracic Society. San Diego, CA, May 16–21, 2014.

19. Rao GA, Mann JR, Shoaibi A, et al. Azithromycin and levofloxacin use and increased risk of cardiac arrhythmia and death. Ann Fam Med 2014;12: 121–7.

20. Koh WJ, Hong G, Kim SY, et al. Treatment of refractory Mycobacterium avium complex lung disease with a moxifloxacin-containing regimen. Antimicrob Agents Chemother 2013;57:2281–5.

21. Jo KW, Kim S, Lee JY, et al. Treatment outcomes of refractory MAC pulmonary disease treated with drugs with unclear efficacy. J Infect Chemother 2014;20(10):602–6.

22. Field SK, Cowie RL. Treatment of Mycobacterium avium-intracellulare complex lung disease with a macrolide, ethambutol, and clofazimine. Chest 2003;124:1482–6.

23. Jarand J, Davis JP, Cowie RL, et al. Long-term follow-up of mycobacterium avium complex lung disease in patients treated with regimens including Clofazimine and/or Rifampin. Chest 2016;149: 1285–93.

24. van Ingen J, Totten SE, Helstrom NK, et al. In vitro synergy between clofazimine and amikacin in treatment of nontuberculous mycobacterial disease. Antimicrob Agents Chemother 2012;56:6324–7.

25. Shen GH, Wu BD, Hu ST, et al. High efficacy of clofazimine and its synergistic effect with amikacin against rapidly growing mycobacteria. Int J Antimicrob Agents 2010;35:400–4.

26. Martiniano SL, Wagner BD, Levin A, et al. Safety and effectiveness of clofazimine for primary and refractory nontuberculous mycobacterial infection. Chest 2017;152:800–9.

27. Yang B, Jhun BW, Moon SM, et al. Clofazimine-containing regimen for the treatment of mycobacterium abscessus lung disease. Antimicrob Agents Chemother 2017;61 [pii:e02052-16].

28. Philley JV, Wallace RJ Jr, Benwill JL, et al. Preliminary results of bedaquiline as salvage therapy for patients with nontuberculous mycobacterial lung disease. Chest 2015;148:499–506.

29. Alexander DC, Vasireddy R, Vasireddy S, et al. Emergence of mmpT5 variants during bedaquiline treatment of mycobacterium intracellulare lung disease. J Clin Microbiol 2017;55:574–84.

30. Brown-Elliott BA, Philley JV, Griffith DE, et al. In vitro susceptibility testing of bedaquiline against mycobacterium avium complex. Antimicrob Agents Chemother 2017;61 [pii:e01798-16].

31. Hartkoorn RC, Uplekar S, Cole ST. Cross-resistance between clofazimine and bedaquiline through upregulation of MmpL5 in Mycobacterium tuberculosis. Antimicrob Agents Chemother 2014;58:2979–81.

32. Winthrop KL, Ku JH, Marras TK, et al. The tolerability of linezolid in the treatment of nontuberculous mycobacterial disease. Eur Respir J 2015;45:1177–9.

33. Wallace RJ Jr, Brown-Elliott BA, Ward SC, et al. Activities of linezolid against rapidly growing mycobacteria. Antimicrob Agents Chemother 2001; 45:764–7.

34. Brown-Elliott BA, Wallace RJ Jr, Blinkhorn R, et al. Successful treatment of disseminated Mycobacterium chelonae infection with linezolid. Clin Infect Dis 2001;33:1433–4.

35. Griffith DE, Brown-Elliott BA, Wallace RJ Jr. Thrice-weekly clarithromycin-containing regimen for treatment of Mycobacterium kansasii lung disease: results of a preliminary study. Clin Infect Dis 2003; 37:1178–82.

36. van Ingen J, Boeree MJ, Dekhuijzen PN, et al. Clinical relevance of Mycobacterium simiae in pulmonary samples. Eur Respir J 2008;31:106–9.

37. Valero G, Moreno F, Graybill JR. Activities of clarithromycin, ofloxacin, and clarithromycin plus ethambutol against Mycobacterium simiae in murine model of disseminated infection. Antimicrob Agents Chemother 1994;38:2676–7.

38. Valero G, Peters J, Jorgensen JH, et al. Clinical isolates of Mycobacterium simiae in San Antonio, Texas. An 11-yr review. Am J Respir Crit Care Med 1995;152:1555–7.

39. Jenkins PA, Campbell IA, Banks J, et al. Clarithromycin vs ciprofloxacin as adjuncts to rifampicin and ethambutol in treating opportunist mycobacterial lung diseases and an assessment of Mycobacterium vaccae immunotherapy. Thorax 2008;63: 627–34.

40. Andrejak C, Lescure FX, Pukenyte E, et al. Mycobacterium xenopi pulmonary infections: a multicentric retrospective study of 136 cases in north-east France. Thorax 2009;64:291–6.

41. van Ingen J, Boeree MJ, de Lange WC, et al. Mycobacterium xenopi clinical relevance and determinants, the Netherlands. Emerg Infect Dis 2008;14: 385–9.

42. Andrejak C, Almeida DV, Tyagi S, et al. Improving existing tools for Mycobacterium xenopi treatment: assessment of drug combinations and characterization of mouse models of infection and chemotherapy. J Antimicrob Chemother 2013;68:659–65.

43. Yoo H, Jeon K, Kim SY, et al. Clinical significance of Mycobacterium szulgai isolates from respiratory specimens. Scand J Infect Dis 2014;46:169–74.

44. van Ingen J, Boeree MJ, de Lange WC, et al. Clinical relevance of Mycobacterium szulgai in The Netherlands. Clin Infect Dis 2008;46:1200–5.

45. Tortoli E, Kohl TA, Brown-Elliott BA, et al. Mycobacterium abscessus, a taxonomic puzzle. Int J Syst Evol Microbiol 2018;68:467–9.

46. Leao SC, Tortoli E, Euzeby JP, et al. Proposal that Mycobacterium massiliense and Mycobacterium bolletii be united and reclassified as Mycobacterium abscessus subsp. bolletii comb. nov., designation of Mycobacterium abscessus subsp. abscessus subsp. nov. and emended description of Mycobacterium abscessus. Int J Syst Evol Microbiol 2011; 61:2311–3.

47. Tortoli E, Kohl TA, Brown-Elliott BA, et al. Emended description of Mycobacterium abscessus, Mycobacterium abscessus subsp. abscessus and Mycobacteriumabscessus subsp. bolletii and designation of Mycobacteriumabscessus subsp. massiliense comb. nov. Int J Syst Evol Microbiol 2016;66:4471–9.

48. Adekambi T, Sassi M, van Ingen J, et al. Reinstating Mycobacterium massiliense and Mycobacterium bolletii as species of the Mycobacterium abscessus complex. Int J Syst Evol Microbiol 2017;67:2726–30.

49. Tan JL, Ngeow YF, Choo SW. Support from Phylogenomic Networks and Subspecies Signatures for Separation of Mycobacterium massiliense from Mycobacterium bolletii. J Clin Microbiol 2015;53: 3042–6.

50. Nash KA, Brown-Elliott BA, Wallace RJ Jr. A novel gene, erm(41), confers inducible macrolide resistance to clinical isolates of Mycobacterium abscessus but is absent from Mycobacterium chelonae. Antimicrob Agents Chemother 2009;53:1367–76.

51. Koh WJ, Jeon K, Lee NY, et al. Clinical significance of differentiation of Mycobacterium massiliense from Mycobacterium abscessus. Am J Respir Crit Care Med 2011;183:405–10.

52. Jeon K, Kwon OJ, Lee NY, et al. Antibiotic treatment of Mycobacterium abscessus lung disease: a retrospective analysis of 65 patients. Am J Respir Crit Care Med 2009;180:896–902.

53. Choi GE, Shin SJ, Won CJ, et al. Macrolide treatment for Mycobacterium abscessus and Mycobacterium massiliense infection and inducible resistance. Am J Respir Crit Care Med 2012;186:917–25.

54. Jarand J, Levin A, Zhang L, et al. Clinical and microbiologic outcomes in patients receiving treatment for Mycobacterium abscessus pulmonary disease. Clin Infect Dis 2011;52:565–71.

55. Wallace RJ Jr, Dukart G, Brown-Elliott BA, et al. Clinical experience in 52 patients with tigecycline-containing regimens for salvage treatment of Mycobacterium abscessus and Mycobacterium chelonae infections. J Antimicrob Chemother 2014; 69:1945–53.

56. Koh WJ, Jeong BH, Kim SY, et al. Mycobacterial characteristics and treatment outcomes in mycobacterium abscessus lung disease. Clin Infect Dis 2017;64:309–16.

57. Lee H, Sohn YM, Ko JY, et al. Once-daily dosing of amikacin for treatment of Mycobacterium abscessus lung disease. Int J Tuberc Lung Dis 2017;21:818–24.

58. Choi H, Jhun BW, Kim SY, et al. Treatment outcomes of macrolide-susceptible Mycobacterium abscessus lung disease. Diagn Microbiol Infect Dis 2018; 90:293–5.

59. Turenne CY, Tschetter L, Wolfe J, et al. Necessity of quality-controlled 16S rRNA gene sequence databases: identifying nontuberculous Mycobacterium species. J Clin Microbiol 2001;39:3637–48.

60. Patel JB, Leonard DG, Pan X, et al. Sequence-based identification of Mycobacterium species using the MicroSeq 500 16S rDNA bacterial identification system. J Clin Microbiol 2000;38:246–51.

61. Flume PA, Robinson KA, O'Sullivan BP, et al. Cystic fibrosis pulmonary guidelines: airway clearance therapies. Respir Care 2009;54:522–37.

62. Lester MK, Flume PA. Airway-clearance therapy guidelines and implementation. Respir Care 2009; 54:733–50 [discussion: 751–3].

63. Donaldson SH, Bennett WD, Zeman KL, et al. Mucus clearance and lung function in cystic fibrosis with hypertonic saline. N Engl J Med 2006;354:241–50.

64. Elkins MR, Robinson M, Rose BR, et al. A controlled trial of long-term inhaled hypertonic saline in patients with cystic fibrosis. N Engl J Med 2006;354: 229–40.

65. Snijders D, Fernandez Dominguez B, Calgaro S, et al. Mucociliary clearance techniques for treating non-cystic fibrosis bronchiectasis: is there evidence? Int J Immunopathol Pharmacol 2015;28: 150–9.

66. Nicolson CH, Stirling RG, Borg BM, et al. The long term effect of inhaled hypertonic saline 6% in non-cystic fibrosis bronchiectasis. Respir Med 2012; 106:661–7.

67. Kellett F, Robert NM. Nebulised 7% hypertonic saline improves lung function and quality of life in bronchiectasis. Respir Med 2011;105:1831–5.

68. O'Donnell AE, Barker AF, Ilowite JS, et al. Treatment of idiopathic bronchiectasis with aerosolized recombinant human DNase I. rhDNase Study Group. Chest 1998;113:1329–34.

69. Bilton D, Tino G, Barker AF, et al. Inhaled mannitol for non-cystic fibrosis bronchiectasis: a randomised, controlled trial. Thorax 2014;69:1073–9.

70. Feazel LM, Baumgartner LK, Peterson KL, et al. Opportunistic pathogens enriched in showerhead biofilms. Proc Natl Acad Sci U S A 2009;106: 16393–9.

71. Falkinham JO 3rd. Nontuberculous mycobacteria from household plumbing of patients with nontuberculous mycobacteria disease. Emerg Infect Dis 2011;17:419–24.

72. Falkinham JO 3rd, Iseman MD, de Haas P, et al. Mycobacterium avium in a shower linked to pulmonary disease. J Water Health 2008;6:209–13.

73. Wallace RJ Jr, Iakhiaeva E, Williams MD, et al. Absence of Mycobacterium intracellulare and presence of Mycobacterium chimaera in household water and biofilm samples of patients in the United States with Mycobacterium avium complex respiratory disease. J Clin Microbiol 2013;51:1747–52.

74. Nishiuchi Y, Maekura R, Kitada S, et al. The recovery of Mycobacterium avium-intracellulare complex (MAC) from the residential bathrooms of patients with pulmonary MAC. Clin Infect Dis 2007;45: 347–51.

75. Fujita K, Ito Y, Hirai T, et al. Association between polyclonal and mixed mycobacterial Mycobacterium avium complex infection and environmental exposure. Ann Am Thorac Soc 2014;11:45–53.

76. Lee AL, Hill CJ, Cecins N, et al. The short and long term effects of exercise training in non-cystic fibrosis bronchiectasis–a randomised controlled trial. Respir Res 2014;15:44.

Surgical Treatment of Pulmonary Nontuberculous Mycobacterial Infections

John D. Mitchell, MD

KEYWORDS

- Bronchiectasis • Thoracoscopic lobectomy • VATS lobectomy • Thoracoscopic segmentectomy
- VATS segmentectomy • Nontuberculous mycobacteria

KEY POINTS

- Adjuvant surgical resection for patients with pulmonary nontuberculous mycobacterial (NTM) infection can be accomplished with acceptable morbidity and mortality and leads to a high culture conversion rate.
- Resection of bronchiectasis or cavitary lung disease associated with pulmonary NTM disease is often feasible through a minimally invasive surgical approach, with excellent outcomes.
- Bronchopleural fistula remains a troubling complication following pneumonectomy for pulmonary NTM infection, particularly on the right side.
- Consideration of adjuvant surgical resection for pulmonary NTM disease is best approached in experienced centers, with a committed multidisciplinary team of clinicians involved.

INTRODUCTION

Although the actual figures remain elusive, most clinicians believe that the incidence of pulmonary nontuberculous mycobacterial (NTM) disease is increasing in North America and is significantly more common than lung infection due to *Mycobacterium tuberculosis*. Although targeted antimicrobial therapy remains the mainstay of therapy in these patients, failure of medical therapy is not uncommon. Reasons for treatment failure (beyond drug resistance, intolerance, or lack of access) include the presence of parenchymal lung damage in the form of severe bronchiectasis or cavitary lung disease. The addition of *adjunctive* surgical resection has been used to improve treatment success rates in those with focal parenchymal damage such as bronchiectasis or cavitary lung disease. The rationale for adding surgery to the treatment of affected patients is that these areas of parenchymal disease are poorly penetrated by the antibiotic therapy and thus serve as a "reservoir" for organisms to trigger recurrent infection. In this article, the common indications, techniques, and outcomes of pulmonary NTM surgery are discussed.

INDICATIONS FOR SURGERY

The indications for surgery are listed in **Box 1**. All patients must have met the criteria for pulmonary NTM infection described in the American Thoracic Society guidelines,[1] have focal parenchymal disease amenable to resection, and possess adequate pulmonary reserve in light of the planned surgical procedure. Only a minority of patients who

Disclosures: The author has nothing to disclose.
Section of General Thoracic Surgery, Division of Cardiothoracic Surgery, University of Colorado School of Medicine, Academic Office 1, Room 6602, C-310, 12631 East 17th Avenue, Aurora, CO 80045, USA
E-mail address: john.mitchell@ucdenver.edu

Thorac Surg Clin 29 (2019) 77–83
https://doi.org/10.1016/j.thorsurg.2018.09.011

> **Box 1**
> **Indications for surgery in pulmonary nontuberculous mycobacterial disease**
>
> 1. Failure of medical therapy
>   Recurrent infection
>   Antibiotic resistance
>   Antibiotic intolerance
> 2. Symptom control
> 3. Limit disease progression

can alleviate these symptoms even if residual disease (typically, bronchiectasis) remains. Finally, in a small subset of cases, "debulking" of the most severe parenchymal damage may limit or slow down disease progression; in these patients, it is recognized that surgery is unlikely to produce even temporary eradication of the infection, but may slow disease extension to less affected areas. An example of this latter category would be a patient with severe unilateral cavitary disease with less parenchymal change on the contralateral side.

present with NTM infection will be eligible for resection.

Three main indications for surgery exist.[2] In most cases, resectional surgery is performed after failure of medical therapy, as a means to induce treatment success. In these cases, the parenchymal disease should be truly "focal" in nature, whereby following resection the remaining lung is relatively free of structural damage. Often, patients exhibit recurrent treatment failures, often in the setting of antimicrobial resistance. In other patients, the main indication for surgical intervention is to reduce or eliminate troubling or potentially life-threatening symptoms, such as hemoptysis or a chronic, persistent cough. Surgical resection

PREOPERATIVE EVALUATION

Surgery for NTM pulmonary disease is used only as part of a multimodality treatment approach. At our institution, patients appropriate for surgical therapy are discussed at a weekly multidisciplinary conference attended by surgeons, pulmonologists, and infectious disease clinicians with specialization in mycobacterial disease.

Surgical patients usually present with 1 of 3 main patterns of disease. The first, so-called "Lady Windermere syndrome" is characterized by right middle lobe and lingular bronchiectasis and is seen almost exclusively in women (**Fig. 1**). These patients undergo staged thoracoscopic resections about 6 weeks apart, after antibiotic

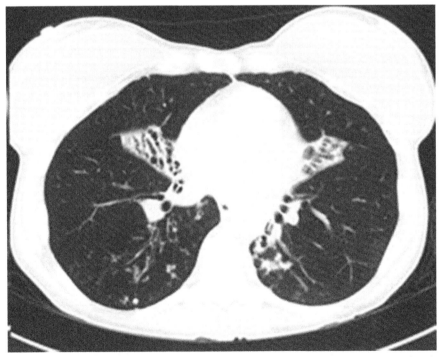

Fig. 1. Computed tomographic image of right middle lobe and lingular bronchiectasis associated with pulmonary NTM disease—the so-called "Lady Windermere syndrome."

pretreatment.[3] The second pattern of presentation involves focal bronchiectasis (**Fig. 2**) or cavitary lung disease (**Fig. 3**). If focal, surgical excision is offered after an appropriate duration of targeted antimicrobial therapy. Occasionally, one may present with bilateral combinations of bronchiectasis and cavitary disease. Although it is tempting to surgically address the most severe side first, we often surgically target the lesser side first to allow for a thoracoscopic approach to both sides. For example, a patient with a right upper lobe cavity and right middle lobe and lingular bronchiectasis would have a thoracoscopic lingulectomy, followed by a right upper and middle bilobectomy; if the bilobectomy were done first, the patient might not tolerate one lung anesthesia to remove the lingula. The third common presentation involves complete lung destruction leading to pneumonectomy (**Fig. 4**).

Patient referrals undergo an extensive assessment at our hospital, including sputum analysis, radiologic, and physiologic testing. High-resolution computed tomography of the chest is performed to assess the extent of the parenchymal lung disease and to assess feasibility of a minimally invasive approach.[4] Adequate pulmonary reserve is assured using pulmonary function testing, with occasional use of perfusion scanning and exercise testing when appropriate. Bronchoscopy is performed when appropriate, primarily for diagnostic purposes and to rule out concomitant endobronchial pathology. In the setting of active hemoptysis, bronchoscopy is used to localize the source within the bronchial tree to the segmental or even subsegmental level. Collection of sputum and bronchoalveolar lavage specimens allows identification of the likely microbial pathogens. Evaluation of culture results

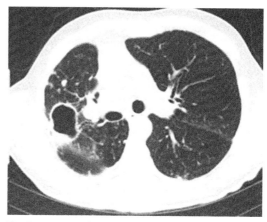

Fig. 3. Computed tomographic image of isolated cavitary lung disease.

includes in-vitro susceptibility testing appropriate for the cultured organism. Patients are then typically initiated on 3- or 4-drug oral antimicrobial therapy, often combined with intravenous or inhaled antibiotics as indicated. Revisions to the planned therapy are occasionally made due to intolerance to the initial regimen. The duration of the preoperative antibiotic therapy varies but typically lasted 8 to 12 weeks for NTM infections. If an adequate regimen was established before presentation, the time delay to surgical intervention can be accelerated. The goal with the preoperative therapy is to achieve a "nadir" in the mycobacterial counts before surgical resection, which is thought to help minimize perioperative complications.

A complete nutritional assessment was made at the time of initial presentation, and dietary supplementation was initiated when indicated. Feeding tubes were generally felt to be unnecessary in these patients with limited, focal parenchymal disease. In addition, all patients were evaluated for the presence of significant gastroesophageal reflux. If present and thought to be a contributing

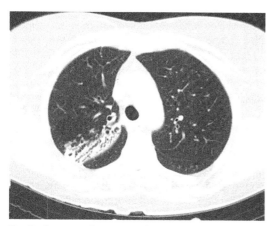

Fig. 2. Computed tomographic image of focal bronchiectasis of the posterior segment of the right upper lobe.

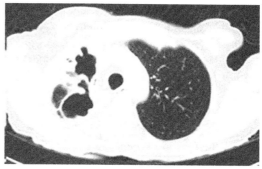

Fig. 4. Computed tomographic image of severe cavitary disease leading to complete lung destruction.

factor to the patient's chronic pulmonary disease, recommendations were made for possible antireflux surgery with or soon after pulmonary resection.

After the planned duration of preoperative antibiotic therapy, patients returned for repeat clinical and radiologic evaluation before surgery. Computed tomography scanning again confirmed the presence of focal disease amenable to surgical resection. Occasionally, isolated cavities may close with intensified medical therapy, thus lessening the need for resection. Assessment of pulmonary function is made if not done previously to ensure adequate postoperative pulmonary reserve in view of the planned resection. Nutritional status is again evaluated and consultation with nutritional specialists obtained as indicated. Careful attention is paid to other known or potential comorbidities in this patient population and addressed as needed.

ANESTHETIC CONSIDERATIONS

Epidural catheters are offered to all patients undergoing an open procedure or in cases where the feasibility of a minimally invasive approach is unknown. Intercostal blocks are used in thoracoscopic cases. The use of a double-lumen tube is standard for airway management; in some cases, ventilation is optimized with initial bronchoscopy and pulmonary toilet maneuvers. In addition, bronchoscopy may allow for identification of variations in normal bronchial anatomy, particularly important in segmentectomy cases. Arterial line monitoring is used selectively. Other standard maneuvers such as deep vein thrombosis (DVT) and antibiotic prophylaxis are used.

SURGICAL TECHNIQUE

Open operations are performed through a lateral thoracotomy incision, with harvest of the latissimus dorsi muscle or intercostal muscle if planned. The previous incision is used in the case of reoperation. For cases of completion or extrapleural pneumonectomy where extensive extrapleural dissection would be used, the fifth or sixth rib is usually removed to facilitate exposure and help define the extrapleural plane. Our techniques used in completion pneumonectomy have been previously described.[5]

There are numerous differences between anatomic resection for lung cancer and for mycobacterial disease. Adhesions are typically found throughout the opened hemithorax, particularly involving the diseased lung segments. These adhesions are divided with blunt dissection, the cautery, or other energy device, taking care to identify

and preserve vital structures. The bronchial circulation is hypertrophied and without care can obscure tissue planes and cause considerable blood loss during hilar dissection. Lymph nodes within the hilum are numerous and enlarged and at times can be densely adherent to the adjacent structures, complicating the dissection. Fissures may be fused due to the long-standing inflammatory state. Vital structures, such as the phrenic nerve, may be obscured by the same process, making identification and preservation difficult. These differences are often neglected by the occasional NTM surgeon, who applies the more familiar oncologic techniques and principles during the procedure, leading to a suboptimal outcome. As with any complex surgical technique, these patients are usually best served by referral to centers with considerable experience in this infectious lung surgery. Anatomic lung resection (segmentectomy, lobectomy, and pneumonectomy) is preferred to minimize postoperative complications and to ensure complete resection of the involved area.

However, once these factors are accounted for, the planned anatomic resection may be then carried out using standard techniques. The pulmonary vessels are ligated with a vascular stapling device. The bronchi are closed with either an Endo GIA stapler (Medtronic, Inc, Dublin, Ireland) or with interrupted absorbable suture. The fissures and lines of parenchymal division for segmentectomy are completed using the Endo-GIA stapler, taking care to completely excise the involved, diseased lung.

Ideally, the removed specimens are "double cultured" with samples sent to 2 separate microbiology laboratories to minimize sampling error. After placement of chest drains, routine techniques are used to close the incision. Blood loss is usually minimal except in cases of totally destroyed lung, extensive extrapleural dissection, or in the reoperative setting.

Most of our NTM cases are now completed using minimally invasive (video-assisted thoracoscopic surgery [VATS]) techniques. The authors' preliminary experience with this approach has been reported previously.[6] Two 10 mm ports and a 3 cm "utility" incision are used, the latter covered with a wound protector. In cases of *Mycobacterium abscessus*, where the risk of wound infection is increased, all ports should be covered with wound protectors. No rib spreading was used. The resection was otherwise carried out in an identical fashion to the open approach. Most of these patients have focal bronchiectasis or cavitary lung disease and have a manageable degree of pleural symphysis. With experience, the surgeon can readily identify most cases amenable to a VATS approach; in some patients, exploratory thoracoscopy may be needed to demonstrate feasibility of a minimally invasive approach. In the authors' experience, much depends on the perseverance of the surgeon.

In patients with mycobacterial infection, the residual lung is often poorly compliant and fails to "fill" the remaining space within the ipsilateral hemithorax. If the residual space is considerable, the authors occasionally used autologous tissue and/or limited thoracoplasty to reduce it. Indications for muscle transposition included not only issues of residual space but also to buttress the bronchial closure. This latter approach was used frequently (although not routinely) in cases of pneumonectomy or particularly poorly controlled infection at the time of operation. Latissimus dorsi or intercostal muscle was used for this purpose and is amenable to harvest through minimally invasive techniques. Use of the serratus anterior muscle is poorly tolerated in this characteristically thin patient population due to the resulting winged scapula that results from the muscle harvest. In severe cases, an omental pedicle may be used to buttress the bronchial closure after pneumonectomy. The omental harvest is typically performed by the same thoracic team and completed via limited upper midline abdominal incision just before the thoracotomy. The technique of omental transposition has been previously reported.[7]

In patients with overt pleural space involvement due to perforation or large, thin-walled cavitary disease where the risk of spillage is great during resection (**Fig. 5**), preoperative counseling is performed regarding open thoracostomy. The authors' usual practice is to pack the hemithorax with dilute Dakin's solution daily, followed by a

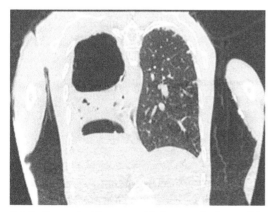

Fig. 5. Computed tomographic image of a large, thin walled cavity at risk of disruption and spillage during resection.

Clagett procedure using antibiotic solution 6 to 12 weeks after the initial resection.

POSTOPERATIVE CARE

In general, postoperative care is routine. Preoperative antibiotic regimens are continued throughout the preoperative period and altered (typically with cessation of parenteral medications) within 1 month. Fluids are limited per standard lung resection protocols. DVT and atrial arrhythmia prophylaxis is routine. A strong emphasis is placed on early mobilization and chest physiotherapy. Chest tubes are removed with cessation of air leak and acceptable daily output.

OUTCOMES

Postoperative surgical outcomes following resection for pulmonary NTM disease are outlined in **Table 1**.[3,7–14] These series report acceptable morbidity and mortality (particularly in light of the surgery performed) and a high "culture conversion" rate after the procedure. These data suggest that anatomic resection may be performed safely in these patients and can be efficacious in the treatment of these infections. Readers should be reminded, although, that these are selected patients treated in multidisciplinary environments; similar results are unlikely to be seen when these techniques are applied in an isolated, random fashion.

The authors have previously documented their experience with thoracoscopic resection for patients with pulmonary NTM disease,[3,6] reporting minimal morbidity, no mortality, and hospital stays of just more than 3 days in these selected patients. These outcomes are comparable to those seen with similar resections performed for lung malignancy. As noted earlier, muscle flap transposition is entirely feasible using a thoracoscopic approach. Further studies from other centers are needed to corroborate these findings and provide guidance in proper patient selection.

One troubling but interesting finding in NTM surgery is the high rate of bronchopleural fistula (BPF) after pneumonectomy, particularly on the right side. Mitchell and colleagues[7] reported a 33% rate of BPF after right pneumonectomy, with similar outcomes reported by Shiraishi[15] (60%) and Koh[11] (25%). The fistula rate following pneumonectomy for NTM disease is considerably worse than that seen in patients undergoing similar resection for multidrug-resistant tuberculosis.[16] Poorly controlled infection, significant cavitary disease, and the setting of completion pneumonectomy are felt to be factors in BPF development.

Table 1
Selected series of anatomic resection for pulmonary nontuberculous mycobacterial infection

Author, Year	N	Mortality (%)	Morbidity (%)	BPF (%)	Sputum Conversion (%)
Corpe,[9] 1981	131	6.9	NR	5.3	93
Nelson et al,[12] 1998	28	7.1	32	3.6	88
Watanabe et al,[14] 2006	22	0	NR	NR	95
Koh et al,[11] 2008	23	4.3	35	8.7	100
Mitchell et al,[7] 2008	265	2.6	18.5	4.2	NR
Yu et al,[3] 2011	172	0	7	0	84
Shiraishi et al,[13] 2013	65	0	12	0	100
Kang et al,[10] 2015	70	1.4	21	6.8	81
Asakura et al,[8] 2017	125	3	22	6	91

Abbreviations: BPF, bronchopleural fistula; NR, not reported.

It is possible that aggressive buttressing of the bronchial stump will help mitigate this serious complication.

Data regarding long-term outcomes following adjuvant surgical resection for pulmonary NTM infection remain scarce. Jarand and colleagues[17] compared outcomes in 107 patients receiving treatment for *M abscessus* infection and noted significant improvements in culture conversion and 1-year culture negativity in those treated with adjuvant surgical therapy compared with medical therapy alone (57% vs 28%). Asakura and colleagues[8] reported their long-term outcomes in 125 patients with NTM following adjuvant surgical therapy and found pneumonectomy and residual cavitary disease to be predictors of microbiological recurrence. In the same report, pneumonectomy, low body mass index, old age, and residual cavitary disease were noted on multivariate analysis to be predictors of poor prognosis. More research is needed in this area.

SUMMARY

Adjuvant surgical resection for pulmonary NTM infection can be performed safely and may improve treatment outcomes in selected patients. Many of the procedures are amenable to a minimally invasive surgical approach. Patient selection and preparation are key, and these patients are best served in a multidisciplinary environment with experience in this area. More research is needed regarding long-term outcomes for pulmonary NTM treatment, particularly when adjuvant resection is used.

REFERENCES

1. Griffith DE, Aksamit T, Brown-Elliott BA, et al. An official ATS/IDSA statement: diagnosis, treatment, and prevention of nontuberculous mycobacterial diseases. Am J Respir Crit Care Med 2007;175(4): 367–416.
2. Mitchell JD. Surgical approach to pulmonary nontuberculous mycobacterial infections. Clin Chest Med 2015;36(1):117–22.
3. Yu JA, Pomerantz M, Bishop A, et al. Lady Windermere revisited: treatment with thoracoscopic lobectomy/segmentectomy for right middle lobe and lingular bronchiectasis associated with nontuberculous mycobacterial disease. Eur J Cardiothorac Surg 2011;40(3):671–5.
4. Yen Y-T, Wu M-H, Cheng L, et al. Image characteristics as predictors for thoracoscopic anatomic lung resection in patients with pulmonary tuberculosis. Ann Thorac Surg 2011;92(1):290–5.
5. Sherwood JT, Mitchell JD, Pomerantz M. Completion pneumonectomy for chronic mycobacterial disease. J Thorac Cardiovasc Surg 2005;129(6):1258–65.
6. Mitchell JD, Yu JA, Bishop A, et al. Thoracoscopic lobectomy and segmentectomy for infectious lung disease. Ann Thorac Surg 2012;93(4):1033–9 [discussion: 1039–40].
7. Mitchell JD, Bishop A, Cafaro A, et al. Anatomic lung resection for nontuberculous mycobacterial disease. Ann Thorac Surg 2008;85(6):1887–92 [discussion: 1892–3].
8. Asakura T, Hayakawa N, Hasegawa N, et al. Long-term outcome of pulmonary resection for nontuberculous mycobacterial pulmonary disease. Clin Infect Dis 2017;65(2):244–51.
9. Corpe RF. Surgical management of pulmonary disease due to Mycobacterium avium-intracellulare. Rev Infect Dis 1981;3(5):1064–7.
10. Kang HK, Park HY, Kim D, et al. Treatment outcomes of adjuvant resectional surgery for nontuberculous mycobacterial lung disease. BMC Infect Dis 2015;15:76.
11. Koh WJ, Kim YH, Kwon OJ, et al. Surgical treatment of pulmonary diseases due to nontuberculous mycobacteria. J Korean Med Sci 2008;23(3):397–401.

12. Nelson KG, Griffith DE, Brown BA, et al. Results of operation in Mycobacterium avium-intracellulare lung disease. Ann Thorac Surg 1998;66(2):325–30.

13. Shiraishi Y, Katsuragi N, Kita H, et al. Adjuvant surgical treatment of nontuberculous mycobacterial lung disease. Ann Thorac Surg 2013;96(1):287–91.

14. Watanabe M, Hasegawa N, Ishizaka A, et al. Early pulmonary resection for Mycobacterium avium complex lung disease treated with macrolides and quinolones. Ann Thorac Surg 2006;81(6): 2026–30.

15. Shiraishi Y, Nakajima Y, Katsuragi N, et al. Pneumonectomy for nontuberculous mycobacterial infections. Ann Thorac Surg 2004;78(2):399–403.

16. Shiraishi Y, Katsuragi N, Kita H, et al. Different morbidity after pneumonectomy: multidrug-resistant tuberculosis versus non-tuberculous mycobacterial infection. Interact Cardiovasc Thorac Surg 2010;11(4):429–32.

17. Jarand J, Levin A, Zhang L, et al. Clinical and microbiologic outcomes in patients receiving treatment for Mycobacterium abscessus pulmonary disease. Clin Infect Dis 2011;52(5):565–71.

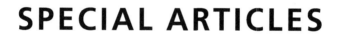

SPECIAL ARTICLES

Mycobacterial Musculoskeletal Infections

John I. Hogan, MD[a], Rocío M. Hurtado, MD, DTM&H[b], Sandra B. Nelson, MD[c],*

KEYWORDS

- *Mycobacterium tuberculosis* • Nontuberculous mycobacteria • Septic arthritis • Pott's disease
- Osteomyelitis • Tenosynovitis

KEY POINTS

- Patients may be predisposed to mycobacterial musculoskeletal infection by virtue of geographic exposure to *Mycobacterium tuberculosis*; cell-mediated immunosuppression, including use of immunomodulatory therapies; or traumatic or postsurgical inoculation of environmental mycobacteria.
- Mycobacteria often cause paucibacillary disease and may be fastidious in their growth characteristics. Diagnosis usually requires culture confirmation but newer molecular technologies offer the potential to identify infecting organisms more rapidly. Sensitivity testing is recommended whenever possible.
- Mycobacterial musculoskeletal infections remain challenging to treat, requiring combination antimycobacterial therapy generally for a minimum of 6 months. Surgical therapy is often required for infection caused by nontuberculous mycobacteria.

INTRODUCTION

Mycobacterial musculoskeletal infections have contributed to significant morbidity for millennia. Researchers have extracted *Mycobacterium tuberculosis* (MTb) DNA from bone lesions of humans who lived more than 9000 years ago.[1] Despite significant advances in modern medicine, these infections remain challenging to manage. Host deficiencies, antibiotic resistance, drug toxicities, limited medication penetration into bone, and complex surgical considerations can all complicate management of these infections. Additional difficulties stem from limited clinical data to guide therapy for patients with severe mycobacterial infections of bones and joints.

This article therefore offers a framework for the approach to musculoskeletal mycobacterial infections, acknowledging that when data are lacking, expert opinion guides much of the management of these infections.

PATHOGENESIS AND HOST RISK FACTORS

Mycobacteria have evolved alongside humans for millennia. Over this period of coevolution, agents of mycobacterial disease have developed a variety of molecular mechanisms that allow them to evade immune detection, avoid destruction within the host, and eventually propagate to effect clinical disease if left unchecked. On initial inhalation, MTb adheres to complement, Fc receptors, and

This article originally appeared in *Infectious Disease Clinics of North America*, Volume 31, Issue 2, June 2017.
Disclosures: None of the authors have any relevant disclosures or financial conflicts of interest.
[a] Division of Infectious Diseases, Massachusetts General Hospital, Harvard Medical School, Cox Building, 5th Floor, 55 Fruit Street, Boston, MA 02114, USA; [b] Mycobacterial Diseases Center, Division of Infectious Diseases, Massachusetts General Hospital, Harvard Medical School, Cox Building, 5th Floor, 55 Fruit Street, Boston, MA 02114, USA; [c] Program in Musculoskeletal Infections, Division of Infectious Diseases, Massachusetts General Hospital, Harvard Medical School, Cox Building, 5th Floor, 55 Fruit Street, Boston, MA 02114, USA
* Corresponding author.
E-mail address: sbnelson@mgh.harvard.edu

thoracic.theclinics.com

mannose receptors present on the surfaces of macrophages.[2] Like other mycobacteria, the initial stage of infection with this pathogen is characterized by an early transition to the intracellular space. MTb and nontuberculous mycobacteria (NTM) actively infect the same cells that are instrumental in their clearance, and on moving into the intracellular space, they avoid detection by other arms of the immune system. Once inside the macrophage, MTb interferes with the expression of various proteins involved in pH regulation and produces a urease that prevents acidification of the phagosome.[2,3] Other NTM adopt a similar strategy.[4] Mycobacteria, including MTb, are also known to express superoxide dismutase, catalase, and thioredoxin to mitigate the reactive oxygen species produced by phagocytic cells.[5] Even if multiple intracellular mechanisms fail to control the intracellular propagation of mycobacteria, macrophage apoptosis mediated by tumor necrosis factor (TNF)–alpha can limit the propagation and viability of mycobacterial species like MTb.[6] However, virulent strains of MTb may still interfere with macrophage apoptosis, thus enhancing their propagation.[7] After becoming established in the intracellular space, cellular immunity becomes essential in clearing mycobacterial infections. TNF-alpha, interleukin (IL)-12, and interferon (IFN)-gamma help to facilitate control of these primarily intracellular pathogens.

Patients with certain inherited and acquired immunodeficiencies or other medical comorbidities are known to be at higher risk of mycobacterial infection in general (**Box 1**). In addition, use of corticosteroids and other immunomodulatory medications has now become one of the most common factors predisposing to invasive mycobacterial disease. In particular, TNF-alpha modulators confer a significant risk of reactivation of tuberculosis, and a growing number of reports suggest that these agents can also increase the risk of invasive NTM infections.[8–10] Although infliximab and adalimumab seem to confer greater risk than etanercept, all three of these immunomodulators may increase the risk of new or reactivated musculoskeletal infections with acid-fast bacilli (AFB).

RISK FACTORS FOR MUSCULOSKELETAL INVOLVEMENT

In a susceptible host, mycobacterial musculoskeletal infections may occur via several different mechanisms. Tuberculosis generally spreads to osteoarticular sites via the hematogenous route. During primary infection with MTb, bacillemia may occur, although it is usually contained by

---

Box 1
Host risk factors for mycobacterial infection

Genetic risks

Mutations that interfere with IFN-gamma production and signaling

Mutations that interfere with IL-12 production and signaling

Mutations that interfere with STAT signaling

MonoMAC syndrome

Chronic granulomatous disease

Acquired immunodeficiencies

Autoantibodies targeting IFN-gamma

Iatrogenic immunosuppression, including corticosteroids and TNF-alpha inhibitors

Medical comorbidities

Human immunodeficiency virus/acquired immunodeficiency syndrome

Malnutrition

Malignancy

Diabetes mellitus

Chronic renal disease

Advanced age

Abbreviations: MonoMAC, monocytopenia and mycobacterial infection; STAT, signal transducer and activator of transcription.

---

cell-mediated immunity. When cellular immunity is impaired, bacillemia may lead to seeding of sanctuary sites, including bones and joints. Osteoarticular tuberculosis may manifest during primary infection, although more commonly it represents reactivation of latent bacilli well after an initial bout of primary disease.

Although osteoarticular infection caused by NTM may occur via hematogenous spread in immunodeficient hosts, contiguous and lymphatic spread of NTM infection after percutaneous inoculation provides another route of infection for NTM. NTM are ubiquitous within the environment, living commensally within soil and water. Traumatic inoculation via environmental vectors (eg, thorns, wood) or via objects contaminated by soil or water can lead to deposition of the organisms within bone or joint spaces. Animal bites and cutaneous injuries in the setting of saltwater exposure have also facilitated serious musculoskeletal infections with mycobacteria.[11–13] Osteoarticular infection associated with injection drug use, in which injection of nonsterile water leads to hematogenous introduction of NTM, has also been reported.[14]

Iatrogenic infections have also occurred. Corticosteroid injections have been associated with outbreaks of NTM infections in joints,[15] presumably caused by contamination of the solution or lack of sterile procedural preparation. Mycobacterial infections may also occur as a consequence of surgery, including those involving prosthetic joints[16] and osteofixation procedures. Cosmetic procedures may also facilitate the inoculation of mycobacteria into skin and soft tissues[17,18] with contiguous spread to adjacent osteoarticular structures. More recently, medical tourism has become a risk factor for invasive mycobacterial disease.[19] Cosmetic procedures performed abroad using suboptimal infection control practices have contributed to disseminated skin and soft tissue mycobacterial infections that may involve bones and joints by contiguous spread.[20] Contamination of irrigant solutions, injectable medications, and surgical instruments may contribute to infection in cases of lipotourism gone awry.[19]

INCIDENCE OF MUSCULOSKELETAL MYCOBACTERIAL INFECTION

Of more than 250,000 patients with tuberculosis reported in the United States between 1993 and 2006, 19% had extrapulmonary disease, of whom 11.3% (2% of all patients with tuberculosis) had osteoarticular involvement.[21] Infections caused by nontuberculous mycobacteria do not require public health reporting, and therefore their exact incidence is not known. More than 120 different species of NTM can cause human infection; the heterogeneity among this diverse group makes these infections challenging to study systematically. For example, between 1965 and 2003, only 31 cases of vertebral osteomyelitis caused by NTM could be identified in the literature.[22] The exact incidence of osteoarticular NTM infections following certain surgical procedures or occurring in specific immunocompromised populations is also not known but is thought to be low.

CLINICAL MANIFESTATIONS
Tuberculosis

Among cases of osteoarticular tuberculosis, the spine is the most commonly affected site of disease. Up to 50% of osteoarticular cases show vertebral involvement[23–25]; this is followed by native septic arthritis primarily involving large joints such as hips and knees. Small joint septic arthritis and osteomyelitis of the extra-axial skeleton occurs less commonly. Multifocal

osteoarticular tuberculosis can also occur.[25] Rarely, tuberculosis may cause prosthetic joint infection.[26] A minority of patients with osteoarticular tuberculosis has concomitant active pulmonary infection. An absence of pulmonary symptoms or radiographic abnormalities should not exclude the diagnosis.

Compared with osteoarticular infections with pyogenic bacteria, infections caused by mycobacteria may present more indolently, evolving over the course of months or even years. Although extracellular pyogenic bacteria effect potent immune activation, mycobacterial infections may elicit a less pronounced initial inflammatory response from the host. In the case of tuberculous septic arthritis, chronic joint effusions and synovitis may be present. When tuberculosis infects prosthetic joints, it typically manifests with pain, swelling, and occasionally drainage from the involved joint. Mycobacterial infections after total knee arthroplasty may become clinically apparent as late as 180 months after arthroplasty.[26] This observation strengthens the hypothesis that MTb infections in prosthetic joints represent latent infection reactivated at the time of surgery. When mycobacterial infections invade deeper osteoarticular structures, a process that initially begins as a synovitis or a periostitis may eventually effect frank erosions of bone. Patients with longstanding infection can eventually develop a significant burden of sequestra and involucra. When liquefied tissue and bone destroyed via caseous necrosis accumulates around a site of infection, a so-called cold abscess may form. Although these collections can contain viable bacilli, they elicit much less inflammation than abscesses containing pyogenic bacteria. When the classic signs of osteoarticular infection are less prominent, other signs and symptoms might raise further suspicion for osteoarticular tuberculosis. Prominent B symptoms, including anorexia, weight loss, fatigue, and night sweats, can all accompany chronic tuberculosis. Regional lymphadenopathy or multiple chronic sinus tracts communicating with bones or joints can also serve as clues.

Spinal osteomyelitis caused by MTb was first described in by Percivall Pott in 1779, and is now commonly referred to as Pott's disease.[27] The anterior portions of the lower thoracic and upper lumbar vertebrae are the most common sites affected by Pott's disease.[28] Although pyogenic bacteria causing vertebral osteomyelitis cause a primary discitis that spreads to adjacent vertebral bodies, MTb classically first infects vertebral bodies. Involvement of the disc space is a later finding, and can be a radiographic clue to the disease. Like other forms of spinal osteomyelitis, Pott's disease may contribute to the development of large paraspinal abscesses. Paraspinal abscesses along the cervical spine may manifest with quadriparesis when compressing the cervical cord or with stridor when compressing the trachea.[23] Pott's disease may be associated with chronic sinus tracts or cold abscesses far removed from the primary site of infection, including the supraclavicular space, the buttocks, and even the popliteal fossa.[2] Despite experiencing frank erosion of bone, patients affected by Pott's disease may lack systemic symptoms, and present only with the insidious onset of gradually worsening back pain. Without treatment, destructive changes contribute to the wedging of adjacent damaged vertebrae, a process that may ultimately culminate in the development of a gibbus deformity. Even after appropriate therapy, deformity may still progress, with many patients experiencing greater than 60° of kyphosis.[29] Neurologic symptoms and true neurologic deficits may occur during the course of disease.[25]

Nontuberculous Mycobacteria

Similar to patients with tuberculosis, patients with musculoskeletal infection caused by NTM may develop subacute to chronic septic arthritis. Vertebral osteomyelitis caused by NTM occurs less commonly than with tuberculosis, and is seen most often in immunocompromised hosts with disseminated infections.[30] NTM also can cause septic tenosynovitis after traumatic inoculation, often in an immunocompetent host. After percutaneous inoculation into soft tissues, NTM may cause a subacute to chronic ulceronodular soft tissue infection that manifests slowly over many months. Although many NTM can cause nodular lymphangitis, the classic syndrome is attributed to *Mycobacterium marinum*, an organism found in saltwater and fishtanks.[31] In chronic soft tissue infection, NTM may extend to involve joints and underlying bone by direct extension. Approximately one-quarter of patients with *M marinum* infection develop tenosynovitis.[32] Although not pathognomonic for tenosynovitis from mycobacterial disease, the presence of so-called rice bodies, white nodules consisting of acidophilic material surrounded by fibrin and collagen embedded within tendon sheaths or bursae, should raise suspicion for the diagnosis.[33] Surgical site infection caused by NTM may manifest with subacute to chronic drainage, multifocal ulceronodular disease, and sinus tracts extending to the deep surgical site.

DIAGNOSIS

Because the treatment of infections caused by mycobacteria require different therapies than those caused by conventional bacterial pathogens, confirming a microbiologic diagnosis is of paramount importance. The diagnosis of mycobacterial musculoskeletal infections may be definite (microbiologically confirmed) or probable (eg, more common in tuberculosis, where there is isolation of mycobacteria at another site, and a concomitant compatible osteoarticular manifestation, with or without compatible histopathology). Attempts at culturing MTb, if successful, provide the additional opportunity for drug-susceptibility testing, which is important given the global distribution of drug resistance. Establishing a microbiologic diagnosis in NTM disease is equally important given the heterogeneity of this group and the differences in susceptibilities to antimicrobials.

Routine laboratory tests are of limited value in diagnosing mycobacterial infection. Abnormal results of noninvasive laboratory assays such as the erythrocyte sedimentation rate and C-reactive protein can increase suspicion for mycobacterial infections of bones and joints. Other noninvasive tests assessing prior exposure to tuberculous antigens, including the purified protein derivative (PPD) test and IFN-gamma release assays (IGRAs), can be helpful, although neither can distinguish between latent and active infection. Further, neither PPD nor IGRA is sensitive or specific enough to make a diagnosis. The absence of positive PPD tests or IGRAs should not exclude a diagnosis of tuberculosis; up to 50% of patients with disseminated tuberculosis have negative PPD tests. However, if either test is positive in a patient presenting with clinical manifestations compatible with osteoarticular tuberculosis, these tests may direct further diagnostics and infection control practices.

Although no single imaging characteristic can definitively differentiate musculoskeletal infections caused by typical pyogenic bacteria from those caused by mycobacteria, radiographic studies can still be important in determining the likelihood of mycobacterial infection. Tuberculous arthritis may be characterized by peripherally located osseous erosions and more gradual narrowing of the joint space than is seen with pyogenic arthritis.[34] Pott's disease has characteristic radiographic features that may help to distinguish it from pyogenic spinal osteomyelitis. These features include multilevel involvement, large paraspinal abscesses, relative sparing of the disc space, and the presence of bone fragments.[34] Angular kyphosis is a later finding. Although plain films may be sufficient to distinguish between pyogenic and tuberculous spinal osteomyelitis in later disease, MRI offers greater sensitivity in early disease and improved resolution of soft tissue findings. MRI may identify rice bodies, providing another clue to mycobacterial infection. Although no single radiographic finding is pathognomonic for mycobacterial infection, MRI and other imaging modalities can be used to characterize the extent of disease and identify structures most heavily affected by infection to guide more invasive diagnostics and source control.

Once suggested by history, laboratory tests, and imaging, more invasive diagnostics are generally required to secure the diagnosis of musculoskeletal mycobacterial infection. Synovial fluid aspiration is the first test of choice for the diagnosis of septic arthritis, although it may not yield a firm diagnosis. Compared with conventional pyogenic arthritis, joints infected with mycobacteria typically yield lower synovial cell counts. One review of 40 patients identified an average leukocyte count of 18,062 cells/μL in patients with tuberculosis arthritis compared with 31,250 cells/μL in joints infected with NTM,[30] both of which are lower than is typically seen in bacterial septic arthritis. In this study, 14% of tuberculous effusions yielded AFB on staining, whereas 25% of the NTM effusions stained positive for AFB.[30] The authors recommend that AFB staining be performed on synovial fluid samples. Although the growth of MTb in culture is optimal to confirm the diagnosis, synovial fluid culture may not yield a diagnosis. One review of 31 cases of large joint effusions caused by tuberculosis showed that cultures of joint aspirates yielded a positive result in 61% of these cases.[30] Similar to cultures of peritoneal and pleural fluid, synovial fluid culture has a lower sensitivity than tissue culture, a finding that underscores the importance of obtaining tissue samples to increase the likelihood of making a diagnosis.

Percutaneous or operative biopsy of synovium, bone, cartilage, or adjacent abscess material offers the best chance of securing a diagnosis. Histology performed on infected tissue obtained from an immunocompetent host often detects either necrotizing or non-necrotizing granulomas, and occasionally yields AFB on staining. However, even the microscopic examination of grossly infected tissue may fail to identify the offending pathogen,[35] and culture of infected tissue remains the gold standard for diagnosis. Because multiple sites may be involved in patients with disseminated tuberculosis and NTM, clinicians may also consider sampling other sources for

mycobacteria, including blood, sputum, urine, and lymph nodes, in an attempt to isolate a mycobacterial pathogen.

Although the morphologic appearance and growth rate of AFB in culture can provide early clues to the identity of the infecting species, final results using conventional methods take longer to provide species-level identification. Rapidly growing NTM may be identified in days, although the isolation and identification of MTb and slow-growing NTM may take up to 8 weeks or longer. Direct nucleic acid amplification may provide more rapid species-level identification and evidence of antimicrobial resistance genes once an organism has grown in the laboratory, although culture remains imperative for sensitivity testing to fully inform antibiotic selections. One group showed that polymerase chain reaction (PCR) correctly identified MTb in soft tissue specimens obtained from 4 joints infected with this pathogen.[35] Another group reported that, using tissue samples from 19 patients with culture-confirmed Pott's disease, PCR had a sensitivity of 94.7% and a specificity of 83.3%.[36] In cases in which mycobacterial infection is suspected but culture results are negative, PCR may be able to identify a pathogen, although without the important benefit of susceptibility results. However, few data are available on the sensitivity and specificity of PCR in the diagnosis of culture-negative tuberculosis, or in osteoarticular infections caused by NTM. Molecular tests may still be useful in the detection of fastidious mycobacteria such as *Mycobacterium genavense*, particularly when conventional mycobacterial culture fails to identify an organism. Given the ubiquity of environmental mycobacteria, and because PCR cannot distinguish between infecting and contaminating organisms, care to exclude specimen contamination before testing is imperative. Molecular probes assessing for the presence of genes that confer resistance to specific antibiotics have the potential to rapidly identify resistant isolates. The GeneXpert nucleic acid amplification assay for rifampin (RIF) resistance in MTb is one of the most commonly used assays of this kind. Although the use of such tests may prove useful, the operating characteristics of these molecular assays have not been thoroughly validated for use in osteoarticular infections.

THERAPY FOR MYCOBACTERIAL MUSCULOSKELETAL INFECTIONS
General Approaches

Once the diagnosis of musculoskeletal mycobacterial infections is suspected or confirmed, medical management should be planned, and surgical management may need to be considered. Although virtually all musculoskeletal mycobacterial infections require medical therapy, some can be managed with close monitoring but without the need for surgery. Care teams consisting of infectious disease specialists, orthopedic surgeons, rheumatologists, and radiologists may work together to determine optimal therapeutic approaches. Because of the potential toxicity of mycobacterial therapy and the potential for drug interactions, a careful understanding of comorbidities and other medications is necessary. For patients receiving immunomodulatory therapy, strong consideration should be given to stopping immunosuppressive medications, particularly TNF-alpha inhibitors, or substituting with less immunosuppressive alternatives. The diagnosis of tuberculosis may also confer important public health and infection control considerations.

Mycobacterium tuberculosis

The initial management of osteoarticular tuberculosis consists of early and effective antitubercular therapy, assessment of complications that may merit additional intervention, and repeated assessments of clinical response over time to assist in determination of the ultimate length of therapy. Initial medical therapy for drug-susceptible tuberculosis consists of a combination of drugs including rifampin (RIF), isoniazid (isonicotinylhydrazine [INH]), pyrazinamide (PZA), and ethambutol (EMB) administered over a period of 2 months[37] (**Table 1**). Of these agents, INH and RIF possess the most potent early antibacillary effect, and should be included in the regimen whenever possible.[23] Antimycobacterial agents achieve sufficient levels within nonsclerotic bone to achieve bactericidal activity against MTb.[38] After the induction period, patients with drug-susceptible disease should continue for an additional 4 to 10 more months of therapy, ideally with INH and RIF depending on clinical and radiographic evolution. During this continuation phase of therapy, RIF becomes especially important in eradicating quiescent bacilli.[23] In patients who cannot tolerate or have isolates resistant to 1 or more of the antimicrobials listed earlier, guidelines are available through the American Thoracic Society (ATS), the Centers for Disease Control and Prevention (CDC), and the Infectious Diseases Society of America (IDSA).[37,39] Expert consultation should guide therapeutic decisions. Some data suggest that therapeutic drug monitoring may optimize clinical outcomes.[40] The authors recommend that, whenever possible, physicians should monitor drug levels to ensure that they are within the therapeutic range for infections in sanctuary sites such as bone, although the direct impact on outcomes remains unknown.

Although the standard antibiotic regimen used to treat susceptible pulmonary tuberculosis is widely accepted, the optimal duration of medical therapy for patients presenting with tuberculous infections of bones and joints is less well defined. Most of the knowledge comes from studies on spinal tuberculosis. One of the first studies to address this question came from the Tenth Report of the Medical Research Council Working Party on Tuberculosis of the Spine.[41] In this 1986 study, 51 patients with Pott's disease underwent excision of diseased bone with placement of bone graft (Hong Kong procedure) followed by 6 months of INH/RIF/streptomycin or the same treatment followed by 3 additional months of INH/RIF. All but 1 of the patients had a favorable clinical outcome at 3 years, suggesting that 9 months of therapy may offer little benefit compared with 6 months. Another trial randomized 256 patients to 1 of 4 treatment groups: 6 months of INH/RIF, 9 months of INH/RIF, 9 months of INH plus either EMB or para-aminosalicylic acid (PAS), or 18 months of INH plus either EMB or PAS.[42] Overall, only 8% of the patients experienced an adverse clinical outcome at 3 years, although the rate was 19% for those receiving 9 months of INH plus either EMB or PAS. This trial suggests that a 6-month course of INH/RIF is adequate for most cases of Pott's disease, although if an alternative regimen (INH plus EMB or PAS) is needed the course should be extended to 18 months. In addition, a 5-year study randomized 451 ambulatory patients with Pott's disease to 6 months of INH/RIF, 9 months of INH/RIF, surgical intervention followed by 6 months of INH/RIF, 9 months of INH plus either EMB or PAS, or 18 months of INH plus either EMB or PAS.[43] After 5 years, only the group that received 9 months of INH plus either EMB or PAS experienced a higher rate of adverse outcomes. These results and others prompt us to treat patients with tuberculous musculoskeletal infections with a minimum of 6 months of potent therapy, preferably containing a backbone of INH/RIF. Therapy may be extended to 9 to 12 months in patients who initially present with a significant burden of disease or when the net state of immunosuppression is high. Treatment courses of 18 months or longer should be considered when INH/RIF cannot be used.

Many cases of spinal tuberculosis can be managed without operative debridement, although the data to guide decisions around surgery are more limited and are based largely on expert opinion. In ambulatory patients, resection

Table 1
Initial antibiotic regimens frequently used for common osteoarticular mycobacterial infections[a]

Species	Drug Regimen
MTb	Rifampin plus isoniazid plus pyrazinamide plus EMB
Mycobacterium avium complex[b]	Rifampin plus (azithromycin or clarithromycin) plus EMB
Mycobacterium kansasii	Rifampin plus isoniazid[c] plus EMB
Mycobacterium marinum	Rifampin plus EMB plus (azithromycin or clarithromycin)
Mycobacterium abscessus	(Clarithromycin or azithromycin)[d] plus amikacin plus (cefoxitin or imipenem)
Mycobacterium fortuitum[e]	Amikacin plus trimethoprim/ sulfamethoxazole plus quinolone
Mycobacterium chelonae	(Clarithromycin or azithromycin) plus tobramycin plus imipenem

[a] Antimicrobial sensitivities and host factors ultimately dictate the choice of therapy. This table outlines some of the antimicrobial regimens frequently used for sensitive isolates (or as empiric therapy if treatment is started before availability of drug-susceptibility testing). Additional information is available in published reatment guidelines.[8,37] Please note that only a few laboratories screen for inducible macrolide resistance (caused by the erm gene) in rapid growers; this may therefore affect the accuracy of macrolide susceptibility results.

[b] If the pathogen is sensitive to amikacin, providers may consider adding this agent to the initial regimen to address severe infections.

[c] Azithromycin and clarithromycin are also active against most isolates. In certain settings, providers may consider substituting azithromycin or clarithromycin for isoniazid. There is controversy regarding the clinical significance of the low-level isoniazid resistance that is sometimes noted in susceptibility testing. All isolates must be tested for rifamycin resistance. Rifamycin sensitivity correlates well with clinical outcomes.

[d] M abscessus isolates other than subspecies massiliense are frequently resistant to macrolides (inducible resistance). If the isolate is known to be resistant to clarithromycin/azithromycin, providers may instead use tigecycline.

[e] Inducible macrolide resistance is common, and therefore macrolides are often not active agents for this infection.

of infected bone and placement of bone graft confers no major advantage over medical therapy alone.[41,43] ATS/CDC/IDSA guidelines suggest surgery should be considered for patients with Pott's disease who have significant neurologic deficits related to cord compression, an unstable spine predisposing to cord injury, and those who do not respond to medical therapy.[37] Although surgery is not always necessary for cure, the role of stabilizing surgery for Pott's disease to decrease long-term spinal deformity remains controversial. Some experts also favor operative intervention in patients with very large abscesses or those with a significant burden of devitalized or sclerotic bone in the spine.[38,44,45]

As in Pott's disease, extra-axial tuberculosis can often be managed with medical therapy alone.[45] Large abscesses and significant devitalized bone should be considered for surgery. In cases of septic arthritis failing medical therapy, debridement may improve functional outcomes. Patients with substantial joint destruction characterized by significant loss of joint space and those with fibrous ankylosis with significant loss of function or chronic pain may also benefit from operative management. Physicians may consider excisional arthroplasty or arthrodesis to improve mobility and minimize chronic discomfort.[45] Optimally, total joint arthroplasty after tuberculosis arthritis should be deferred until patients show no evidence of recurrent disease after completion of therapy given the potential for reactivation disease after arthroplasty.[46] The duration of time necessary to exonerate the potential for reactivation is not known; one author recommends several years off antibiotics before arthroplasty and an additional 3 to 5 months of therapy after arthroplasty to prevent reactivation.[45] Although total joint arthroplasty during the phase of active medical treatment of tuberculosis is not preferred, in some settings it may be unavoidable, and in these cases arthroplasty followed by long-term antimycobacterial therapy may be used with some success.[47]

The surgical management of prosthetic joint infection related to MTb is controversial. The authors recommend that large effusions be drained, and that devitalized tissue and purulence be debrided. Because tuberculosis does not form biofilms to the extent that Staphylococcus and other typical bacterial species do, hardware may be successfully retained in many cases of MTb prosthetic joint infection.[25] Incision and drainage with liner exchange may be sufficient for many cases of prosthetic joint infection caused by MTb. Complicated infections characterized by hardware loosening, exposed hardware, or the formation of a significant burden of involucra or sequestra should prompt providers to consider removing the prosthesis. It is not known whether a 2-stage hardware management strategy offers any benefit compared with a 1-stage exchange in such cases. Expert opinion guides much of the surgical management of complicated prosthetic joint infections related to MTb.

Nontuberculous Mycobacteria

Much of what is known about the management of osteoarticular infections caused by NTM is either derived from case reports and case series or extrapolated from the tuberculosis literature. The ATS and IDSA have published useful general guidelines discussing therapy for these infections.[8] A minimum of 6 months of multidrug therapy guided by antibiotic sensitivities is usually required for treatment of NTM musculoskeletal infection. However, the optimal length of therapy is not known. Factors including disease burden, virulence of the infecting species, efficacy of available antimycobacterial drugs, degree of host immunosuppression, completeness of surgical debridement (when undertaken), and clinical response affect decision making regarding the duration of therapy. Treatment durations of 12 months or longer may be warranted for severe infections. In the case of more resistant pathogens, such as Mycobacterium abscessus, physicians may need to use combination intravenous antibiotics over a prolonged period, and drug toxicity may also contribute to decisions about therapy duration.

In contrast with tuberculosis, osteoarticular infections caused by NTM often require combined medical and surgical management. NTM are intrinsically more resistant to antimycobacterial therapy compared with MTb, and thorough surgical debridement is often necessary for clinical cure. Even with thorough debridement and appropriate medical therapy, infection may recur and necessitate repeated debridement for infection control. In the setting of prosthetic material, successful eradication of NTM infection is unlikely, and hardware removal is recommended to facilitate cure whenever possible. Although there are few case reports describing patients with prosthetic joint infection caused by NTM species successfully treated with hardware retention,[48] the risk of recurrent infection is unknown but is thought to be high. Limited choices for safe long-term suppression of many NTM in the setting of retained hardware further limit this option. Clinicians may consider hardware retention with long-term suppression for less aggressive NTM infections that are sensitive to safe oral antibiotics, although the risk of relapse is unknown and few data exist to guide these decisions.

If prosthetic material is removed, the authors recommend the use of antibiotic-eluting polymethyl methacrylate cement for local delivery of effective antimycobacterial therapy. Many agents active against NTM are thermostable and can be incorporated into cement, including aminoglycosides, some cephalosporins, macrolides, carbapenems, and quinolones.[49] However, the recommended antibiotic doses for cement are based on minimal inhibitory concentrations (MICs) against conventional pyogenic bacteria. As these drugs require higher MICs to target mycobacteria, higher antibiotic doses in cement may be necessary to achieve the desired local tissue concentration. However, the higher antibiotic doses may be offset by loss of stability of the cement, which can lead to fracturing, and the risk of systemic antimicrobial toxicity, particularly with aminoglycosides.[50] Involvement of infectious diseases pharmacists can be particularly useful as antimicrobial selection and dosing for spacers is considered.[51]

SUMMARY

Although less common as causes of musculoskeletal infection than pyogenic bacteria, mycobacterial musculoskeletal infections remain important causes of morbidity worldwide. Although tuberculous arthritis and osteomyelitis have been recognized for millennia, infections caused by NTM are being identified more often, likely because of both a more susceptible host population and improvements in diagnostic capabilities. Infections caused by mycobacteria remain challenging to diagnose, because of the paucibacillary nature of musculoskeletal infection and fastidious growth characteristics. Despite improvements in molecular diagnostic approaches to mycobacterial infection, culture-based diagnosis remains critical for susceptibility testing, which is paramount to guide treatment decisions. The role of surgery in tuberculous arthritis and osteomyelitis is controversial, but many patients with drug-susceptible disease can be cured without surgery. Because of intrinsically greater resistance among NTM, surgical management is usually required for cure. Although modern surgical and medical therapies afford cure in most cases, substantial long-term morbidity may still result. The limited understanding of these complicated infections underscores the need for higher quality data in the future to guide patient care.

REFERENCES

1. Hershkovitz I, Donoghue HD, Minnikin DE, et al. Detection and molecular characterization of 9000-year-old *Mycobacterium tuberculosis* from a Neolithic settlement in the eastern Mediterranean. PLoS One 2008;3(10):e3426.

2. Bennett JE, Dolin R, Blaser MJ, et al. Mandell, Douglas, and Bennett's principles and practice of infectious diseases. 8th edition. Philadelphia: Elsevier/Saunders; 2015.

3. Glickman MS, Jacobs WR Jr. Microbial pathogenesis of *Mycobacterium tuberculosis*: dawn of a discipline. Cell 2001;104(4):477–85.

4. Sturgillkoszycki S, Schlesinger PH, Chakraborty P, et al. Lack of acidification in *Mycobacterium* phagosomes produced by exclusion of the vesicular proton-ATPase. Science 1994;263(5147):678–81.

5. Edwards KM, Cynamon MH, Voladri RK, et al. Iron-cofactored superoxide dismutase inhibits host responses to *Mycobacterium tuberculosis*. Am J Respir Crit Care Med 2001;164:2213–9.

6. Oddo M, Renno T, Attinger A, et al. Fas ligand-induced apoptosis of infected human macrophages reduces the viability of intracellular *Mycobacterium tuberculosis*. J Immunol 1998; 160(11):5448–54.

7. Keane J, Remold HG, Kornfeld H. Virulent *Mycobacterium tuberculosis* strains evade apoptosis of infected alveolar macrophages. J Immunol 2000; 164(4):2016–20.

8. Griffith DE, Aksamit T, Brown-Elliott BA, et al. An official ATS/IDSA statement: diagnosis, treatment, and prevention of nontuberculous mycobacterial diseases. Am J Respir Crit Care Med 2007;175(4): 367–416.

9. Keane J, Gershon S, Wise RP, et al. Tuberculosis associated with infliximab, a tumor necrosis factor alpha-neutralizing agent. N Engl J Med 2001;345: 1098–104.

10. Keane J. Tumor necrosis factor blockers and reactivation of latent tuberculosis. Clin Infect Dis 2004;39: 300–2.

11. Hofer M, Hirschel B, Kirschner P, et al. Brief report: disseminated osteomyelitis from *Mycobacterium ulcerans* after a snakebite. N Engl J Med 1993; 328(14):1007–9.

12. Clark RB, Spector H, Friedman DM, et al. Osteomyelitis and synovitis produced by *Mycobacterium marinum* in a fisherman. J Clin Microbiol 1990; 28(11):2570–2.

13. Earl T. A chigger bite activates a dormant infection in an outdoorsman. J Am Acad Physician Assist 2010; 23(12):1–3.

14. Longardner K, Allen A, Ramgopal M. Spinal osteomyelitis due to *Mycobacterium fortuitum* in a former intravenous drug user. BMJ Case Rep 2013;2013.

15. Jung SY, Kim BG, Kwon D, et al. An outbreak of joint and cutaneous infections caused by non-tuberculous mycobacteria after corticosteroid injection. Int J Infect Dis 2015;36:62–9.

16. Cheung IK, Wilson A. Arthroplasty tourism. Med J Aust 2007;187(11):666–7.

17. Winthrop KL, Abrams M, Yakrus M, et al. An outbreak of mycobacterial furunculosis associated with footbaths at a nail salon. N Engl J Med 2002; 326(18):1366–71.

18. Difonzo EM, Campanile GL, Vanzi L, et al. Mesotherapy and cutaneous *Mycobacterium fortuitum* infection. Int J Dermatol 2009;48(6):645–7.

19. Furuya EY, Paez A, Srinivasan A, et al. Outbreak of *Mycobacterium abscessus* wound infections among "lipotourists" from the United States who underwent abdominoplasty in the Dominican Republic. Clin Infect Dis 2007;46(8):1181–8.

20. Ruegg E, Cheretakis A, Modarressi A, et al. Multisite infection with *Mycobacterium abscessus* after replacement of breast implants and gluteal lipofilling. Case Rep Infect Dis 2015;2015:1–6.

21. Peto HM, Pratt RH, Harrington TA, et al. Epidemiology of extrapulmonary tuberculosis in the United States, 1993–2006. Clin Infect Dis 2009;49(9): 1350–7.

22. Petitjean G, Fluckiger U, Schären S, et al. Vertebral osteomyelitis caused by non-tuberculous mycobacteria. Clin Microbiol Infect 2004;10(11):951–3.

23. Koopman WJ, Moreland LW. Arthritis and allied conditions. 15th edition. Philadelphia: Lippincott Williams & Wilkins; 2005.

24. Rasouli MR, Mirkoohi M, Vaccaro AR, et al. Spinal tuberculosis: diagnosis and management. Asian Spine J 2012;6(4):294–308.

25. Johansen IS, Nielsen SL, Hove M, et al. Characteristics and clinical outcome of bone and joint tuberculosis from 1994 to 2011: a retrospective register-based study in Denmark. Clin Infect Dis 2015; 61(4):554–62.

26. Kim SJ, Kim JH. Late onset *Mycobacterium tuberculosis* infection after total knee arthroplasty: a systematic review and pooled analysis. Scand J Infect Dis 2013;45:907–14.

27. Pott P. The chirurgical works of Percivall Pott, F.R.S., surgeon to St. Bartholomew's Hospital, a new edition, with his last corrections. 1808. Clin Orthop Relat Res 2002;(398):4–10.

28. Gouliamos AD, Kehagias DT, Lahanis S, et al. MRI findings in tuberculous vertebral osteomyelitis: a pictorial review. Eur Radiol 2001;11(4):575–9.

29. Rajasekaran S. The problem of deformity in spinal tuberculosis. Clin Orthop Relat Res 2002;398: 85–92.

30. Shu CC, Wang JY, Yu CJ, et al. Mycobacterial arthritis of large joints. Ann Rhem Dis 2009;68(9): 1504–5.

31. Lam A, Toma W, Schlesinger N. *Mycobacterium marinum* arthritis mimicking rheumatoid arthritis. J Rheumatol 2006;33(4):817–9.

32. Aubry A, Chosidow O, Caumes E, et al. Sixty-three cases of *Mycobacterium marinum* infection: clinical features, treatment, and antibiotic susceptibility of causative isolates. Arch Intern Med 2002;162(15): 1746–52.

33. Lee EY, Rubin DA, Brown DM. Recurrent *Mycobacterium marinum* tenosynovitis of the wrist mimicking extraarticular synovial chondromatosis on MR images. Skeletal Radiol 2004;33(7):405–8.

34. Griffith JF, Kumta SM, Leung PC, et al. Imaging of musculoskeletal tuberculosis: a new look at an old disease. Clin Orthop Relat Res 2002;398:32–9.

35. Dionisios V, Kazakos C, Tilkeridis C, et al. Polymerase chain reaction for the detection of *Mycobacterium tuberculosis* in synovial fluid, tissue samples, bone marrow aspirate and peripheral blood. Acta Orthop Belg 2003;69(5):366–9.

36. Berk RH, Yazici M, Atabey N, et al. Detection of *Mycobacterium tuberculosis* in formaldehyde solution-fixed, paraffin-embedded tissue by polymerase chain reaction in Pott's disease. Spine 1996;21(17):1991–5.

37. Nahid P, Dorman SE, Alipanah N, et al. Official American Thoracic Society/Centers for Disease Control and Prevention/Infectious Diseases Society of America clinical practice guidelines: treatment of drug-susceptible tuberculosis. Clin Infect Dis 2016; 63(7):e147–95.

38. Ge Z, Wang Z, Wei M. Measurement of the concentration of three antituberculosis drugs in the focus of spinal tuberculosis. Eur Spine J 2008;17(11): 1482–7.

39. Treatment of tuberculosis. Centers for Disease Control and Prevention Website. 2003. Available at: http://www.cdc.gov/mmwr/preview/mmwrhtml/rr5211a1.htm. Accessed September 1, 2016.

40. Alsultan A, Peloquin CA. Therapeutic drug monitoring in the treatment of tuberculosis: an update. Drugs 2014;74(8):839–54.

41. A controlled trial of six-month and nine-month regimens of chemotherapy in patients undergoing radical surgery for tuberculosis of the spine in Hong Kong. Tenth report of the Medical Research Council Working Party on Tuberculosis of the Spine. Tubercle 1986;67(4):243–59.

42. Controlled trial of short-course regimens of chemotherapy in the ambulatory treatment of spinal tuberculosis. Results at three years of a study in Korea. Twelfth report of the Medical Research Council Working Party on Tuberculosis of the Spine. J Bone Joint Surg Br 1993;75(2):240–8.

43. Five-year assessment of controlled trials of short-course chemotherapy regimens of 6, 9 or 18 months' duration for spinal tuberculosis in patients ambulatory from the start or undergoing radical surgery. Fourteenth report of the Medical Research Council Working Party on Tuberculosis of the Spine. Int Orthop 1999;23(2):73–81.

44. Liu P, Zhu Q, Jiang J. Distribution of three antituberculous drugs and their metabolites in different parts of pathological vertebrae with spinal tuberculosis. Spine 2011;36(20):E1290–5.

45. Tuli SM. General principles of osteoarticular tuberculosis. Clin Orthop Relat Res 2002;389:11–9.

46. Berbari EF, Hanssen AD, Duffy MC, et al. Prosthetic joint infection due to *Mycobacterium tuberculosis*: a case series and review of the literature. Am J Orthop 1998;27(3):219–27.

47. Neogi DS, Yadav CS, Ashok Kumar, et al. Total hip arthroplasty in patients with active tuberculosis of the hip with advanced arthritis. Clin Orthop Relat Res 2010;468:605–12.

48. Eid AJ, Berbari EF, Sia IG, et al. Prosthetic joint infection due to rapidly growing mycobacteria: report of 8 cases and review of the literature. Clin Infect Dis 2007;45(6):687–94.

49. Citak M, Argenson JN, Masri B, et al. Spacers. J Arthroplasty 2014;29(2 Suppl):93–9.

50. Prink M, Eckoff DG. *Mycobacterium chelonae* infection following a total knee arthroplasty. J Arthroplasty 1996;11(1):115–6.

51. Curtis JM, Sternhagen V, Batts D. Acute renal failure after placement of tobramycin-impregnated bone cement in an infected total knee arthroplasty. Pharmacotherapy 2005;25(6):876–80.

Nontuberculous Mycobacterial Infections in Cystic Fibrosis

Stacey L. Martiniano, MD[a], Jerry A. Nick, MD[b,c],
Charles L. Daley, MD[b,c],*

KEYWORDS

- Cystic fibrosis • Nontuberculous mycobacteria • *Mycobacterium avium* complex
- *Mycobacterium abscessus* complex

KEY POINTS

- Nontuberculous mycobacterial (NTM) lung infections appear to be increasing in patients with cystic fibrosis (CF).
- *Mycobacterium avium* complex and *Mycobacterium abscessus* complex are the most frequently encountered NTM respiratory pathogens in patients with CF in most areas.
- Diagnosis of NTM lung disease in patients with CF generally follows American Thoracic Society and Cystic Fibrosis Foundation guidelines, with an emphasis on evaluating and treating all known comorbidities.
- Therapy for NTM in patients with CF depends on the species, resistance pattern, and extent of disease.
- Optimal management of patients with CF and NTM lung disease requires carefully considered treatment of both conditions.

INTRODUCTION

Nontuberculous mycobacteria (NTM) have emerged as important pathogens in the setting of cystic fibrosis (CF) lung disease. Although historically CF has been considered a fatal disease of childhood, improvements in therapy have resulted in the oldest and healthiest CF population in history. However, as the disease phenotype has changed in response to improved treatment, it appears that susceptibility to NTM has increased.[1–3] This article reviews the epidemiology, diagnosis, treatment, and prevention of NTM lung disease in people living with CF.

EPIDEMIOLOGY

The CF population has an especially high risk for NTM infection and poses unique challenges with regard to diagnosis, treatment, and prevention.[4] Although the NTM isolation rate in the general population in North America ranges from approximately 6 to 22 per 100,000 and the NTM disease rate from 5 to 10 per 100,000,[5] there is a 1000-fold greater prevalence of NTM in respiratory cultures from patients with CF. The reported prevalence of positive NTM cultures and/or NTM disease within various CF patient cohorts or at single centers varies dramatically,[6,7] but in the

This article originally appeared in *Clinics in Chest Medicine*, Volume 37, Issue 1, March 2016.
Disclosures: The authors are supported by the Cystic Fibrosis Foundation Research Development Grant (NICK15R0).
[a] Department of Pediatrics, Children's Hospital Colorado, University of Colorado Denver School of Medicine, 13123 East 16th Avenue, Box B-395, Aurora, CO 80045, USA; [b] Department of Medicine, National Jewish Health, 1400 Jackson Street, Denver, CO 80206, USA; [c] Department of Medicine, University of Colorado Anschutz Medical Campus, 13001 E. 17th Place, Aurora, CO 80045, USA
* Corresponding author. Department of Medicine, National Jewish Health, 1400 Jackson Street, Denver, CO 80206.
E-mail address: daleyc@njhealth.org

thoracic.theclinics.com

largest studies the overall prevalence is 6% to 13%.[1,3,8–12] In a recent review of data from the US CF Patient Registry, the median state prevalence of NTM in patients with CF was 12%, although this ranged from 0% to 28% (**Fig. 1**). Significant spacial clustering of NTM was detected in Wisconsin, Arizona, Florida, and Maryland.[13]

The prevalence of NTM infection appears to be increasing within the CF population,[1–3,9,14–17] as it is in the general population.[18,19] For example, among patients with CF in Israel, NTM infection prevalence increased threefold from 5% in 2003% to 14.5% in 2011.[16] The reasons for the increase in prevalence are uncertain but culture techniques, increased physician awareness, and more frequent diagnosis of "nonclassic" forms of CF in adulthood may contribute to the apparent increase in NTM prevalence observed in this population.[14]

Most NTM species recovered in CF samples in the United States are from either the *Mycobacterium avium* complex (MAC) or the *Mycobacterium abscessus* complex (MABSC).[12] MAC has historically been the most common NTM isolated from respiratory specimens,[20–23] and in the largest US survey it was present in up to 72% of patients with NTM-positive sputum cultures.[9] Among patients with CF in the US Patient Registry during 2010 to 2011, 60% of positive cultures were for MAC, although this ranged by state, from 29% in Louisiana to 100% in Nebraska and Delaware.[12]

The percentage of MABSC reported in patients with CF with NTM-positive sputum cultures has ranged between 16% and 68%,[3,8,9,24] and it appears that the proportion of MABSC is increasing,[1,2,25] with some centers reporting a greater frequency than MAC. In part, this variation may be due to geographic factors, as MABSC appears especially prevalent in Europe,[3,8,24,25] and *Mycobacterium simiae* and MABSC are the most common species isolated in Israel.[16,26] Differences in relative prevalence of MAC and MABSC may also relate to the age of the cohorts studied, as MAC is more often associated with older patients with CF, often diagnosed in adulthood, whereas MABSC is frequently seen in younger patients and those with more severe lung disease.[3,27]

Less frequently isolated species include *Mycobacterium kansasii*[7,8,21,23] and *Mycobacterium fortuitum*.[8,22,28,29]

Individual Risk Factors for Nontuberculous Mycobacteria in Cystic Fibrosis

Our understanding of individual risk factors for NTM in patients with CF is incomplete, as most reports have studied relatively small cohorts from

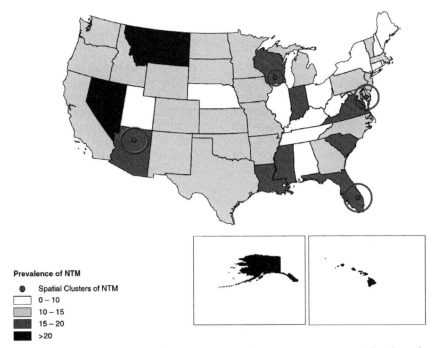

Fig. 1. State-level prevalence and significant (*P*<.05) clusters of NTM among patients with cultured cystic fibrosis, 2010 to 2011. (*Reprinted with* permission of the American Thoracic Society. Copyright © 2015 American Thoracic Society. *From* Adjemian J, Olivier KN, Prevots DR. Nontuberculous mycobacteria among patients with cystic fibrosis in the United States: screening practices and environmental risk. Am J Respir Crit Care Med 2014;190:581–6. The American Journal of Respiratory and Critical Care Medicine is an official journal of the American Thoracic Society.)

single centers or specific geographic areas, often leading to contradictory conclusions. The largest population studies have reported that the increased prevalence of NTM isolation[2,9,10,22,25,26] and NTM disease[26,28] is strongly linked to older age and relatively milder lung disease.[9] A very high prevalence has been reported in adult patients with a "nonclassic" form of CF resulting from residual function mutations.[20,30,31] It is worth noting, however, that other studies have reported the opposite conclusions, in particular that NTM is common in severe lung disease.[10,26,28,32] For example, in Israel, NTM infection was associated with a known "severe" Cystic Fibrosis Transmembrane Conductance Regulator (CFTR) genotype and pancreatic insufficiency.[16]

The presence of Aspergillus fumigatus[2,16,26,33–35] and allergic bronchopulmonary aspergillosis (ABPA)[16,36,37] have been associated with increased risk for NTM. Coinfection with Pseudomonas aeruginosa has been associated with decreased prevalence of NTM in some studies,[9,23] and higher rates of P. aeruginosa coinfection in others.[26] These divergent findings may relate in part to differences in study methodology, as many reports have not distinguished between a positive NTM culture and the presence of NTM disease, and often MAC and MABSC are combined within both adult and pediatric populations.

Although increased survival may indirectly result in greater NTM prevalence through longer cumulative exposure,[38] a greater concern is the possibility that various medications and CF treatment strategies have contributed to the apparent increase in NTM prevalence within this population. Although these reports are not entirely consistent in their conclusions, they have served to heighten awareness of the potential for unforeseen consequences of many therapies in common use. In particular, administration of systemic steroids, often in the context of ABPA treatment, has been associated with increased prevalence of NTM,[26,34,36,37] as well as high-dose ibuprofen.[26] However, other studies have failed to see an increase in NTM-positive cultures with steroid use,[10,26,39] or even an association with decreased NTM.[40]

Use of azithromycin, an antibiotic with anti-inflammatory properties, also has been associated with an increased,[26,41] decreased,[42] or unchanged prevalence of NTM.[39,43,44] Likewise, higher use of antipseudomonal antibiotics has been linked to increased NTM in some,[7,26] but not all reports.[27]

Environmental Risk Factors

Atmospheric conditions appear to explain more of the variation in NTM disease prevalence than individual behaviors in patients with CF in the United States.[45] Among patients with CF at 21 geographically diverse CF centers in the United States, average annual atmospheric water vapor content was significantly predictive of center prevalence ($P = .0019$). The only individual risk factor associated with incident infection was indoor swimming (odds ratio [OR] 5.9, 95% confidence interval [CI] 1.3–26.1). In a review of the prevalence of NTM in the US Patient Registry, high saturated vapor pressure was associated with an increased risk for NTM (OR 1.06, 95% CI 1.02–1.1).[12]

DIAGNOSIS OF NONTUBERCULOUS MYCOBACTERIA LUNG DISEASE IN CYSTIC FIBROSIS

Given the ubiquitous nature of NTM, isolation of an NTM from a respiratory specimen is not synonymous with disease, nor is it necessarily an indication to initiate treatment. Current American Thoracic Society and Infectious Diseases Society of America (ATS/IDSA) criteria for the diagnosis of NTM lung disease calls for the presence of 2 or more positive cultures, in the setting of characteristic clinical symptoms and radiographic findings, and the exclusion of other diseases.[4] These guidelines have not been validated in any patient population, and are particularly challenging in the setting of CF, where radiographic signs suggestive of NTM are common, and identical clinical symptoms can occur due to the near universal presence of coinfections with virulent pathogens, such as P aeruginosa and Staphylococcus aureus.[14]

The primary clinical question for a patient who has cultured positive for a species of NTM on more than one occasion is whether this represents an indolent infection, or actual NTM disease, which may benefit from treatment. Patients who are smear-positive for NTM are more likely to have NTM disease,[23,26] as well as those who demonstrate progression by computed tomography (CT) of the chest of typical findings associated with NTM.[40] Unfortunately, many of the radiographic findings consistent with NTM infection are nonspecific, such as nodules and centrilobular nodules with a tree-in-bud appearance (**Fig. 2**). The presence of cavitation is the most important radiographic finding, as it is a reflection of tissue destruction (**Fig. 3**).

Unexpectedly rapid decline in lung function, specifically, forced expiratory volume in 1 second (FEV_1), is frequently associated with NTM disease in patients with positive cultures for NTM.[28,46,47] In a recent retrospective study, the cohort of patients with NTM disease demonstrated a mean decline in FEV_1 for a year before initial recovery of NTM in

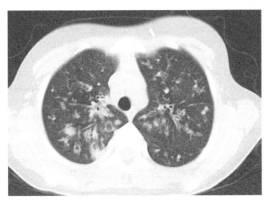

Fig. 2. Radiographic findings of NTM disease in CF. The patient is an 11-year-old with CF and history of chronic *Pseudomonas* infection. In addition, he has had multiple cultures that were positive for *M abscessus* subspecies *abscessus*. Despite several courses of prolonged intravenous, oral, and inhaled drugs he remained culture positive. The CT shows diffuse bronchiectasis, airway wall thickening, extensive mucus plugging, and scattered nodules including centrilobular nodules with a tree-and-bud appearance. The patient had a positive acid-fast smear at the time of this CT.

their sputum.[48] Whereas patients with indolent infection, or patients who apparently cleared the infection after a single positive culture demonstrated a stable FEV$_1$ for a year before, and 3 years

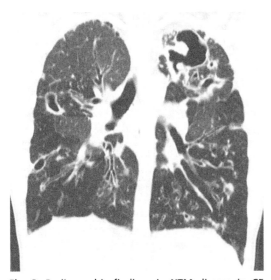

Fig. 3. Radiographic findings in NTM disease in CF. The patient is a 33-year-old diagnosed with CF as an adult. After several years of multidrug therapy for *M avium* complex, the isolate developed macrolide resistance. The CT shows a large left upper lobe cavity with additional smaller cavitary lesions on the right. Note the airways running into the smaller cavities.

after, the initial positive culture.[48] Suggested criteria for the diagnosis of NTM disease in CF is outlined in **Box 1**.[49]

Laboratory Identification of Nontuberculous Mycobacteria in the Cystic Fibrosis Sputum

Historically, descriptions of NTM infection in patients with CF were relatively uncommon,[10,21,22] in part due to the lack of laboratory methodology specific to CF. Recovery of NTM from CF sputum samples was difficult because of culture overgrowth by *P aeruginosa* and other CF microbes before the slower-growing mycobacteria could be detected.[50–52] Development of effective sample decontamination protocols to remove conventional bacteria and fungi has allowed for improved culture-based detection of mycobacteria in CF samples.[53,54]

Currently, the standard approach to decontamination involves 2 steps[51] to avoid excessive decontamination, which can reduce NTM viability in samples.[55] Decontamination is first performed with N-Acetyl L-cysteine-NaOH, before mycobacterial culture.[51,53,54,56] Samples that remain contaminated can then be treated with 5% oxalic acid or alternatively 1% chlorhexidine, which may permit recovery of NTM, although with reduced sensitivity.[50,56–58] A recent study reported the use of a novel culture medium for rapidly growing mycobacteria (RGM) in patients with CF that does not require decontamination.[59] Of 118 isolates of RGM, all but one grew on the agar. RGM were recovered from 54 sputum samples using the RGM media compared with only 17 samples using the control agar.

Both liquid and solid media are recommended for culturing NTM with incubation for at least 6 weeks.[56] Once NTM has been detected in culture, it is critical that the organism is properly speciated, as treatment varies depending on the species. New methods of rapid specification are available, including line probe assays, partial gene sequencing, multilocus sequencing, and matrix-assisted laser desorption ionization-time-of-flight (MALDI-TOF) mass spectrometry. Line probe assays are easy to perform and allow identification of the most frequently encountered NTM; however, these assays are unable to distinguish the different subspecies of MABSC.[60] Partial sequencing allows a higher level of discrimination than line probe assays but requires access to sequencing facilities: 16S rRNA allows discrimination to the species level for most species, whereas *hsp*65, *rpo*B genes, and the 16S-23S internal transcribed spacer allow discrimination to the subspecies level. Sequencing of multiple loci allows

---

Box 1
Suggested criteria for the diagnosis of nontuberculous mycobacteria (NTM) disease in cystic fibrosis (CF)

All 3 criteria should be met before treatment.

1. Positive acid-fast bacilli cultures on at least 2 separate occasions, from either sputum or bronchoalveolar lavage.

2. Clinical, spirometric, and radiographic findings consistent with NTM infection. At least 1 must be present, including

   - Unexplained loss in lung function
   - Increased respiratory symptoms (cough, sputum production, dyspnea, hemoptysis)
   - Constitutional symptoms such as fever, fatigue, night sweats, or weight loss
   - Progression of radiographic features consistent with NTM infection (cavitary disease, single or multiple nodules, tree-in-bud opacities, parenchymal consolidation)

3. Exclusion of other comorbidities common in CF, including adequate treatment of

   - Coinfections, such as *Pseudomonas aeruginosa* and *Staphylococcus aureus*
   - Airway clearance therapy
   - Nutritional deficiencies
   - CF-related diabetes
   - Reactive airway disease and allergic bronchopulmonary aspergillosis
   - CF sinus disease

---

excellent discrimination of the various MABSC subspecies. MALDI-TOF mass spectrometry is a new tool for NTM identification but cannot provide the level of subspecies discrimination given by sequencing.[61]

Drug Susceptibility Testing

The ATS, IDSA, and the Clinical and Laboratory Standards Institute (CLSI) have published recommendations for drug susceptibility testing of the most commonly encountered NTM.[4,62] Except in a few instances, the laboratory-defined cutoffs for resistance have not been validated clinically.

In the setting of MAC infections, resistance to macrolides has been associated with poor clinical outcomes, so current recommendations are to perform susceptibility testing on all initial isolates.[4,62] In addition, repeat testing should be performed if there is failure to convert the culture to negative after 6 months of treatment, when MAC is recultured after completion of treatment (recurrence), or when MAC is recultured after conversion while on treatment (failure).[56]

For RGM, microdilution methods are recommended, although there are no studies that have associated minimum inhibitory concentration (MIC) breakpoints with clinical outcomes in the setting of pulmonary infections.[62] Antimicrobials that should be tested against RGM are amikacin,

tobramycin (for *Mycobacterium chelonae*), cefoxitin, ciprofloxacin, clarithromycin, doxycycline (or minocycline), imipenem, linezolid, moxifloxacin, and trimethoprim-sulfamethoxazole.[62]

Some RGM (*Mycobacterium fortuitum*, *Mycobacterium abscessus* subspecies *abscessus*, and *Mycobacterium abscessus* subspecies *bolettii*) contain an erythromycin resistance methylase (*erm*) gene that causes inducible resistance to macrolides.[63] It is currently recommended that the final reading for macrolide resistance be at least 14 days after inoculation unless resistance (MIC $\geq$8 μg/mL) is noted earlier.[62] Alternatively, molecular identification of a complete, functional gene versus a truncated, nonfunctional gene can be performed.

SCREENING FOR NONTUBERCULOUS MYCOBACTERIA IN THE CYSTIC FIBROSIS POPULATION

NTM are often first detected in a CF sputum sample in the absence of clinical suspicion, as part of routine screening; the optimal frequency for such screening is not known. Among patients with CF 12 years of age or older in the US CF Patient Registry, 58% had mycobacterial cultures of which 14% were positive.[12] Not all of these individuals had NTM lung disease, as small quantities of NTM from the environment may intermittently be present in the CF airway, but not result in NTM pulmonary disease.[9,40,48] Cultures for NTM should be performed annually in spontaneously expectorating patients with a stable clinic course. In the absence of clinical features suggestive of NTM pulmonary disease in individuals unable to spontaneously produce sputum, screening is not required.[56]

Screening also may be considered in several other situations, such as before the initiation of chronic macrolide therapy,[14,40] which has been associated with increased development of resistance to the antibiotic.[64,65] Screening more than once a year also may be considered in various patients deemed to be at higher risk for acquiring the infection, or in which the infection could have more severe consequences. In particular, older patients, those with advanced lung disease awaiting transplantation, and those with previous NTM-positive cultures. Conversely, in small children and individuals not capable of producing a sputum sample, and with no recognized risk factors or clinical symptoms, NTM screening can be deferred.

Nearly all studies reporting prevalence of NTM in the CF population have used acid-fast bacilli (AFB) smear and culture from sputum, either induced or spontaneously produced. Although NTM can, on occasion, be detected through laryngeal suction, oropharyngeal swabs, or gastric aspirate,[21,28,34,66] these methods have not been validated for NTM detection. The use of oropharyngeal swabs is not recommended.[56] Skin testing for delayed-type hypersensitivity against NTM antigens does not appear sufficiently sensitive or specific to use for screening.[21,29,67]

In the future, it is likely that culture-independent methods of NTM detection will be used. In particular, molecular techniques can be performed rapidly, and are extremely sensitive and specific for the detection of NTM in sputum,[68–70] although not yet validated in the setting of CF. Use of serologic assays, such as immunoglobulin (Ig)G against *Mycobacterium* antigen A60 for NTM surveillance appear promising,[71,72] but currently lack validation in the CF population. A recent study from Sweden reported that anti-MABSC IgG ELISA was sixfold higher in patients with CF with MABSC pulmonary disease compared with those without disease: the sensitivity of the assay was 95% and the specificity was 73%.[73]

TREATMENT OF NONTUBERCULOUS MYCOBACTERIA LUNG DISEASE

Treatment of NTM pulmonary disease in CF should be based on ATS/IDSA guidelines that were developed for the general population,[4] as well as guidelines developed under the sponsorship of the US CF Foundation (CFF) and the European CF Society specific to individuals with CF.[56]

Treatment of Mycobacterium avium Complex Lung Disease

Initial treatment for noncavitary NTM disease due to MAC uses a macrolide, rifamycin, and ethambutol.[4] Frequently, azithromycin is the macrolide chosen due to better tolerance, a long history of use in CF lung disease, and fewer interactions with rifampicin and other drugs metabolized through the CYP3A enzyme system compared with clarithromycin.[74] Although azithromycin has recently been shown to reduce macrophage autophagy of *M abscessus*,[41] this potential detriment has not been evaluated in patients with NTM disease. Additionally, chronic azithromycin therapy has been shown to have benefits in people with CF felt to be due to immunomodulatory properties of the drug, in particular those patients with *P aeruginosa*.[75–78]

Intermittent oral antibiotic therapy (ie, 3 times weekly) is recommended for non–CF-related MAC lung disease with less extensive disease and recent studies have demonstrated success rates similar to daily therapy but with less drug intolerance.[79,80] However, intermittent therapy is not recommended in CF due to the presence of underlying lung disease and concerns of reduced absorption of antimycobacterials and altered pharmacokinetics in CF.[56,81]

To date, only the presence of resistance to macrolides has been shown to correlate with worse clinical outcomes.[4] In non CF patients with macrolide-resistant MAC lung disease was associated with a very low culture conversion rate.[65] Surgical resection and use of injectable aminoglycosides for more than 6 months increased the culture conversion rate to 79% from 5%. In patients with CF with MAC that is macrolide-resistant, or who are systemically ill, are AFB smear positive, or have evidence of a cavitary lesion on chest imaging, a 1-month to 3-month course of intravenous daily amikacin may be added at the beginning of the treatment course along with the standard 3 oral antibiotics. Patients within this category should generally be managed in collaboration with an expert in the treatment of NTM disease and CF.

Treatment of Mycobacterium abscessus Complex Lung Disease

Typically, treatment regimens for MABSC are divided into an initial intensive phase followed by a continuation phase. The intensive phase consists of 3 to 12 weeks of 3 antibiotics, including intravenous amikacin, cefoxitin, imipenem, or tige-cycline, in addition to oral antibiotics.[56] After intra-venous therapy, patients usually continue on prolonged chronic suppressive therapy with oral and inhaled treatments with adjustments of therapy based on microbiologic, clinical, and radiographic responses.[82] In some patients, inter-mittent courses of intravenous antibiotics are required to control the infection. Changes to the drug regimen are common, due to patient toler-ance, side effects, and lack of efficacy (**Fig. 4**). These patients also should be generally managed in collaboration with an expert in the treatment of NTM disease and CF.

MABSC can be divided into 3 subspecies, including *M abscessus*, *Mycobacterium bolettii*, and *Mycobacterium massiliense*.[83] *M abscessus* subspecies *abscessus* and subspecies *bolettii* contain an *erm*[41] gene, which can result in induc-ible macrolide resistance. *M massiliense* has a truncated nonfunctional gene so the organism does not develop inducible macrolide resistance. There are significant differences in treatment out-comes for *M abscessus* subspecies *abscessus* and subspecies *massiliense* in both patients with CF and without CF. In a study from France, clarithromycin-based regimens led to mycobacte-rial eradication in 100% of patients with *M massi-liense* but only 27% of patients with *M abscessus* (*P* = .009).[84] These differences are presumably related to the development of inducible macrolide resistance in subspecies *abscessus* but not in *massiliense*. Whether a macrolide should be continued in the face of potential inducible resis-tance is not known, but given the potential immu-nomodulatory benefits in CF lung disease, most providers maintain the macrolide in the treatment regimen.

Monitoring of Drug Toxicity and Clinical Response

Routine monitoring of drug toxicity is essential, and a plan for monitoring should be set in place at the initiation of treatment. Patients with CF are commonly treated with aminoglycosides for other lung pathogens, and therefore prone to auditory-vestibular toxicity and renal injury, making baseline and regular audiology evaluations and monitoring of renal function essential. Even among oral agents, the potential for drug-related side effects and toxicity is considerable, including bone marrow suppression, hepatitis, and QT prolonga-tion. Of particular concern is change in visual acu-ity due to ethambutol. Patients are recommended to monitor their vision daily and the drug should be discontinued immediately at the first sign of vision disturbance.[49]

Therapeutic Drug Monitoring

Recommended dosages of antimycobacterials are based on pharmacokinetic (PK) and pharma-codynamic (PD) data from healthy volunteers and patients with tuberculosis. In patients with non-CF NTM disease, 48% of patients had low serum concentrations of ethambutol, 56% for clarithromycin, and 35% for azithromycin, despite using ATS/IDSA recommended doses.[74] In one small case-series, researchers demon-strated that serum levels of oral agents for the treatment of NTM are usually far below the target range in patients with CF and in one case in which treatment was failing, increasing the dose to achieve therapeutic levels was associ-ated with eradication of the organism.[81] Based on these studies and others, it appears that the dosing of patients with both CF and non-CF NTM disease may in some cases be

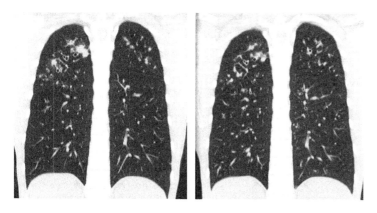

Fig. 4. Treatment response to *M abscessus* subspecies *abscessus*. A 21-year-old with history of previous diagnosis and treatment of *M avium* complex and *Pseudomonas* infections. Despite several rounds of intravenous antimycobacterial therapy, he remained culture positive. He was placed on a "sup-pressive" regimen of inhaled amikacin, clofazimine, and clari-thromycin and his CT scan was repeated after 1 year. The CT scan on the left shows upper lobe pre-dominate bronchiectasis with mucus plugging and nodules. Follow-up CT 1 year later shows that the nodules had diminished in size but he remained culture positive. His spirometric values remained stable.

subtherapeutic, possibly contributing to poor response to treatment.[81]

Challenges to optimal dosing of patients with CF include malabsorption of drug, impaired gastric motility, larger volume of distribution, increased metabolic rate, and potentially increased elimination.[85–87] In addition, drug-drug interactions may occur among various medications used to treat NTM; in particular, rifampin may increase the metabolism of macrolides and moxifloxacin.[74,88] Currently, it is standard practice to monitor amikacin serum levels when administered intravenously. Although sufficient evidence is not available to recommend routine drug monitoring in all patients with CF, it should be considered in the setting of treatment failure, or when multiple drug interactions are possible.[89] In all patients with CF, it must be emphasized that currently available antibiotics have significant limitation in achieving bacteriostatic concentrations within mucus plugs lodged in the airway,[90] thus intensive airway clearance is an essential component of treatment.

NONPHARMACOLOGIC TREATMENT OPTIONS

In addition to pharmacologic treatment of NTM infection, nonpharmacologic therapies for underlying CF lung disease that primarily target clearance of airway mucus obstruction are essential. All NTM treatment regimens need to be part of a comprehensive CF care plan that includes effective airway clearance, nutrition management, and treatment of CF comorbidities, such as sinus disease and CF-related diabetes. This care is most effectively delivered at a CF Care Center, which uses a multidisciplinary approach, providing access to a respiratory therapist, dietitian, and social worker, in addition to nurses and physicians experienced in CF care. The CF Care Centers can be located at http://www.cff.org/LivingWithCF/CareCenterNetwork/CFFoundation-accreditedCareCenters/.

SURGICAL TREATMENT OPTIONS

Surgical resection (pneumonectomy, lobectomy, or segmentectomy) may be a consideration as adjuvant therapy to medical treatment of NTM pulmonary disease. Patients with MABSC lung disease but without CF have been reported to have a higher rate of sustained culture conversion after surgery than with antimicrobial therapy alone.[91,92] In patients with CF, often there is a lobe with a greater burden of disease; however, disease is generally diffuse and bronchiectasis eventually will involve all lobes. It is difficult to identify, with certainty, a focus of NTM infection in the setting of coinfection with typical CF pathogens, such as *P aeruginosa* and *S aureus*, and patients with CF with a history of NTM are at very high risk to acquire a second NTM in their lifetime (**Fig. 5**).[48] In rare circumstances, a patients with CF with NTM disease may be identified who is a good candidate to benefit from lung resection, but only in combination with intensive preoperative and postoperative medical treatment, and in the hands of an experienced thoracic surgeon.[4,93,94]

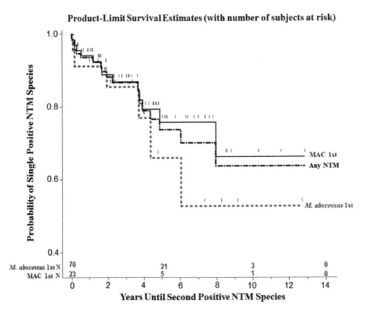

Fig. 5. Probability of detecting a second NTM species after culturing a first NTM. Following an initial positive culture, 24% of subjects with MAC initially grew a second NTM species during 5 years of follow-up, whereas 34% with *M abscessus* first grew a second NTM species at 5 years. Overall, 26% of subjects grew a second NTM species at 5 years and 36% at 10 years. Kaplan-Meier analysis, separated by initial positive NTM culture species. (*Reprinted with* permission of the American Thoracic Society. Copyright © 2014 American Thoracic Society. *From* Martiniano SL, Sontag MK, Daley CL, et al. Clinical significance of a first positive nontuberculous mycobacteria culture in cystic fibrosis. Ann Am Thorac Soc 2014;11:36–44.)

TREATMENT OUTCOMES AND IMPACT OF NONTUBERCULOUS MYCOBACTERIA LUNG DISEASE

Treatment success is generally defined by sustained culture conversion for at least 12 months.[4,92] Rates of successful therapy appear to vary dramatically, based on NTM species, patterns of antibiotic resistance, and severity of disease, as seen in prospective trials in patients with NTM lung disease. In a recent retrospective review of patients with CF from Colorado, the rate of sustained culture conversion in response to initial treatment of MABSC (subspecies not designated) was 45%, and response to treatment of MAC was 60%.[48] The issue of treatment failure is particularly problematic in the context of CF. General considerations in the evaluation of treatment failure include antibiotic resistance, inadequate dosing, and/or poor absorption of antibiotics, suboptimal airway clearance, lack of adherence to the prescribed medications, and the contribution of other comorbidities, including exacerbations of other chronic infections, chronic aspiration, and CF-related diabetes.

RECOMMENDATIONS FOR FOLLOW-UP

After a person with CF has been identified as having a positive NTM culture, close surveillance is warranted, with repeat sputum cultures obtained regularly.[4] Additionally, people with CF with clinical decline or radiographic progression of lung disease that is unresponsive to treatment of typical CF pathogens should be evaluated for NTM. This is particularly important in patients previously infected with an NTM or treated for NTM pulmonary disease, as the presence of a second NTM is a relatively common occurrence. Many previous trials have noted the presence of individuals with more than one species of NTM recovered from their sputum.[1,2,9,22,25–27,95] In patients from the Colorado CF center, we found that MAC was typically the first identified NTM, but a subsequent positive culture for M abscessus was common, whereas subjects who first cultured M abscessus also had a high rate of secondary positive cultures for MAC.[48] Remarkably, 26% of subjects were identified with a second NTM species at 5 years and 36% at 10 years (see **Fig. 5**). These findings support the need for lifelong strategies for NTM surveillance and management in patients with CF who present with a positive NTM culture.

LUNG TRANSPLANTATION IN CYSTIC FIBROSIS AND NONTUBERCULOUS MYCOBACTERIA

Bilateral lung transplantation is an option considered by patients with CF who develop severe bronchiectasis and end-stage lung disease, generally described as an FEV_1 consistently below 30% predicted, a rapid decline in FEV_1, or presence of increased frequency or severity of pulmonary exacerbations.[96] In 2006, the International Society for Heart and Lung Transplantation included colonization with highly resistant or highly virulent bacteria, fungi, or mycobacteria in the list of relative contraindications for lung transplantation.[97]

NTM-positive cultures and NTM pulmonary disease have been reported at a higher prevalence in patients with CF referred for lung transplantation compared with patients without CF.[32] Case reports of death due to disseminated M abscessus after lung transplantation in adult and pediatric patients with CF have been described in people with pretransplant infection,[98–100] although several patients have been described in whom preexisting NTM was not detected but then was a source of posttransplant morbidity and mortality.[99,101,102]

Investigators from the University of North Carolina described a 19.7% prevalence rate of NTM isolated from respiratory cultures from patients with CF referred for transplantation.[32] After transplantation, NTM disease prevalence was low, but a cause of significant morbidity, although no increase in mortality. In a follow-up study, the center reported 13 patients between 1992 and 2012 with at least one pretransplant culture positive for M abscessus (6 were smear positive).[103] Three patients developed M abscessus–related complications with clearance of the organism following treatment. Survival after transplantation was 77% at 1 year, 64% at 3 years, and 50% at 5 years. None of the patients died from M abscessus.

A group from Denmark reviewed 52 patients with CF who underwent lung transplantation, describing a 21% prevalence of NTM-positive cultures pretransplantation and a 17% prevalence of pretransplant NTM pulmonary disease.[104] With perioperative medical treatment, 67% of their patients were alive at follow-up and no deaths had been attributed to NTM infection; however, morbidity, including wound infections, was described. Wound infections from M abscessus posttransplantation also have been reported from Sweden in patients with CF with pretransplant M abscessus.[102]

Based on these studies, it is currently recommended that infection with NTM, even M abscessus, should not be an absolute contraindication to lung transplantation, although morbidity is to be expected.[56] Consensus opinion is that aggressive and prolonged courses of multiple antimycobacterial agents before transplantation, perioperatively, and after transplantation are critical to improving outcomes in these patients.[99,105] The decision to proceed with lung transplantation in patients with active MABSC disease should be made individually by each transplant program; currently most programs decline to perform the transplant under this circumstance.

INFECTION PREVENTION

Infections with NTM have historically been thought to be from environmental exposure[8,106]; however, recently, the potential for patient-to-patient spread within CF centers has been described[95,107–109] with devastating consequences.[109] Five patients who had overlapping clinical encounters at the University of Washington CF Center were found to have identical isolates of M abscessus subspecies massiliense by PFGE (pulsed-field gel electrophoresis) and repetitive unit-sequence–based polymerase chain reaction pattern.[109] In the United Kingdom, another group used whole-genome sequencing as well as analysis of antibiotic resistance patterns to identify 2 clustered outbreaks of M abscessus subspecies massiliense.[108] Both groups suspected indirect person-to-person spread within the clinic and hospital setting. On the other hand, a recent report from the United Kingdom could not demonstrate cross-transmission of M abscessus within a cohort of pediatric patients with CF except between one sibling pair.[110]

Based on these recent reports, the CF Foundation recommends that all health care personnel implement contact precautions (ie, wear a gown and gloves) when caring for all people with CF, regardless of respiratory culture results, in both ambulatory and inpatient settings.[111] Additionally, they recommend that molecular typing of all NTM isolates be performed if there is a suspected patient-to-patient transmission event.

SUMMARY/DISCUSSION

The prevalence of pulmonary NTM infections appears to be increasing in patients living with CF and, based on current trends, it seems likely that NTM infections will continue to increase. The steady improvement in survival achieved over the past 2 decades will likely lead to a greater proportion of the CF population resembling the phenotype best suited to MAC infection; those with less severe CFTR mutations and greater age. Likewise, it appears that the prevalence of MABSC is increasing possibly due to patient-to-patient transmission and that children and patients with more severe pulmonary disease are at risk.

Diagnosis of NTM disease in the setting of CF can be difficult given the overlapping clinical and radiographic findings caused by common CF pathogens and because isolation of NTM may or may not be associated with progressive disease. As treatment may not be necessary in all cases, CF-specific diagnostic criteria are greatly needed.

Treatment presents a significant burden on the patient and health care system,[112] requiring a prolonged multidrug regimen, often including several months of multiple intravenous antibiotics and associated with frequent drug-related toxicities. For patients with CF, this treatment burden comes in addition to existing time-intensive and cost-intensive regimens of medications and airway clearance. Given the increasing common morbidity caused by NTM disease, a significant investment in NTM-related research will be required over the next decades.

REFERENCES

1. Roux A-L, Catherinot E, Ripoll F, et al, Jean-Louis Herrmann for the OMAG. Multicenter study of prevalence of nontuberculous mycobacteria in patients with cystic fibrosis in France. J Clin Microbiol 2009; 47:4124–8.
2. Esther CR Jr, Esserman DA, Gilligan P, et al. Chronic Mycobacterium abscessus infection and lung function decline in cystic fibrosis. J Cyst Fibros 2010;9:117–23.
3. Qvist T, Pressler T, Hoiby N, et al. Shifting paradigms of nontuberculous mycobacteria in cystic fibrosis. Respir Res 2014;15:41.
4. Griffith DE, Aksamit T, Brown-Elliott BA, et al. An official ATS/IDSA statement: diagnosis, treatment, and prevention of nontuberculous mycobacterial diseases. Am J Respir Crit Care Med 2007;175: 367–416.
5. Prevots DR, Marras TK. Epidemiology of human pulmonary infection with nontuberculous mycobacteria: a review. Clin Chest Med 2015;36:13–34.
6. Andre E, Degraux J, Simon A, et al. Absence of non-tuberculous mycobacteria recovery in sputum of cystic fibrosis patients despite adequate decontamination: a possible role of specific antimicrobial therapy used in our centre. Clin Microbiol Infect 2010;16:S33–4.
7. Torrens JK, Dawkins P, Conway SP, et al. Nontuberculous mycobacteria in cystic fibrosis. Thorax 1998;53:182–5.
8. Sermet-Gaudelus I, Le Bourgeois M, Pierre-Audigier C, et al. Mycobacterium abscessus and children with cystic fibrosis. Emerg Infect Dis 2003;9:1587–91.
9. Olivier KN, Weber DJ, Wallace RJ Jr, et al, Nontuberculous Mycobacteria in Cystic Fibrosis Study Group. Nontuberculous mycobacteria. I: multicenter prevalence study in cystic fibrosis. Am J Respir Crit Care Med 2003;167:828–34.

10. Aitken ML, Burke W, McDonald G, et al. Nontuberculous mycobacterial disease in adult cystic fibrosis patients. Chest 1993;103:1096–9.

11. Valenza G, Tappe D, Turnwald D, et al. Prevalence and antimicrobial susceptibility of microorganisms isolated from sputa of patients with cystic fibrosis. J Cyst Fibros 2008;7:123–7.

12. Adjemian J, Olivier KN, Prevots DR. Nontuberculous mycobacteria among patients with cystic fibrosis in the United States: screening practices and environmental risk. Am J Respir Crit Care Med 2014;190:581–6.

13. Adjemian J, Olivier KN, Seitz AE, et al. Spatial clusters of nontuberculous mycobacterial lung disease in the United States. Am J Respir Crit Care Med 2012;186(6):553–8.

14. Leung JM, Olivier KN. Nontuberculous mycobacteria in patients with cystic fibrosis. Semin Respir Crit Care Med 2013;34:124–34.

15. Qvist T, Gilljam M, Jonsson B, et al, Scandinavian Cystic Fibrosis Study Consortium (SCFSC). Epidemiology of nontuberculous mycobacteria among patients with cystic fibrosis in Scandinavia. J Cyst Fibros 2015;14:46–52.

16. Bar-On O, Mussaffi H, Mei-Zahav M, et al. Increasing nontuberculous mycobacteria infection in cystic fibrosis. J Cyst Fibros 2015;14:53–62.

17. Raidt L, Idelevich EA, Dubbers A, et al. Increased prevalence and resistance of important pathogens recovered from respiratory specimens of cystic fibrosis patients during a decade. Pediatr Infect Dis J 2015;34:700–5.

18. Adjemian J, Olivier KN, Seitz AE, et al. Prevalence of nontuberculous mycobacterial lung disease in U.S. Medicare beneficiaries. Am J Respir Crit Care Med 2012;185:881–6.

19. Prevots DR, Shaw PA, Strickland D, et al. Nontuberculous mycobacterial lung disease prevalence at four integrated health care delivery systems. Am J Respir Crit Care Med 2010;182:970–6.

20. Rodman DM, Polis JM, Heltshe SL, et al. Late diagnosis defines a unique population of long-term survivors of cystic fibrosis. Am J Respir Crit Care Med 2005;171:621–6.

21. Hjelte L, Petrini B, Kallenius G, et al. Prospective study of mycobacterial infections in patients with cystic fibrosis. Thorax 1990;45:397–400.

22. Kilby JM, Gilligan PH, Yankaskas JR, et al. Nontuberculous mycobacteria in adult patients with cystic fibrosis. Chest 1992;102:70–5.

23. Esther CR Jr, Henry MM, Molina PL, et al. Nontuberculous mycobacterial infection in young children with cystic fibrosis. Pediatr Pulmonol 2005;40:39–44.

24. Seddon P, Fidler K, Raman S, et al. Prevalence of nontuberculous mycobacteria in cystic fibrosis clinics, United Kingdom, 2009. Emerg Infect Dis 2013;19:1128–30.

25. Pierre-Audigier C, Ferroni A, Sermet-Gaudelus I, et al. Age-related prevalence and distribution of nontuberculous mycobacterial species among patients with cystic fibrosis. J Clin Microbiol 2005;43:3467–70.

26. Levy I, Grisaru-Soen G, Lerner-Geva L, et al. Multicenter cross-sectional study of nontuberculous mycobacterial infections among cystic fibrosis patients, Israel. Emerg Infect Dis 2008;14:378–84.

27. Catherinot E, Roux AL, Vibet MA, et al, OMA Group. *Mycobacterium avium* and *Mycobacterium abscessus* complex target distinct cystic fibrosis patient subpopulations. J Cyst Fibros 2013;12:74–80.

28. Fauroux B, Delaisi B, Clement A, et al. Mycobacterial lung disease in cystic fibrosis: a prospective study. Pediatr Infect Dis J 1997;16:354–8.

29. Hjelt K, Hojlyng N, Howitz P, et al. The role of mycobacteria other than tuberculosis (MOTT) in patients with cystic fibrosis. Scand J Infect Dis 1994;26:569–76.

30. Keating CL, Liu X, Dimango EA. Classic respiratory disease but atypical diagnostic testing distinguishes adult presentation of cystic fibrosis. Chest 2010;137:1157–63.

31. Nick JA, Chacon CS, Brayshaw SJ, et al. Effects of gender and age at diagnosis on disease progression in long-term survivors of cystic fibrosis. Am J Respir Crit Care Med 2010;182:614–26.

32. Chalermskulrat W, Sood N, Neuringer IP, et al. Nontuberculous mycobacteria in end stage cystic fibrosis: implications for lung transplantation. Thorax 2006;61:507–13.

33. Burgel P, Morand P, Audureau E, et al. Azithromycin and the risk of nontuberculous mycobacteria in adults with cystic fibrosis. Pediatr Pulmonology 2011;46:328.

34. Ager S, O'Brien C, Spencer DA, et al. A retrospective review of non-tuberculous mycobacteria in paediatric cystic fibrosis patients at a regional centre. J Cyst Fibros 2011;10:S36.

35. Paugam A, Baixench M-T, Demazes-Dufeu N, et al. Characteristics and consequences of airway colonization by filamentous fungi in 201 adult patients with cystic fibrosis in France. Med Mycol 2010;48(Suppl 1):S32–6.

36. Mussaffi H, Rivlin J, Shalit I, et al. Nontuberculous mycobacteria in cystic fibrosis associated with allergic bronchopulmonary aspergillosis and steroid therapy. Eur Respir J 2005;25:324–8.

37. Evans JT, Ratnaraja N, Gardiner S, et al. *Mycobacterium abscessus* in cystic fibrosis: what does it all mean? Clin Microbiol Infect 2011;17:S602.

38. Falkinham JO 3rd. Surrounded by mycobacteria: nontuberculous mycobacteria in the human environment. J Appl Microbiol 2009;107:356–67.

39. Giron RM, Maiz L, Barrio I, et al. Nontuberculous mycobacterial infection in patients with cystic fibrosis: a multicenter prevalence study. Arch Bronconeumol 2008;44:679–84 [in Spanish].

40. Olivier KN, Weber DJ, Lee J-H, et al, Nontuberculous Mycobacteria in Cystic Fibrosis Study Group. Nontuberculous mycobacteria. II: nested-cohort study of impact on cystic fibrosis lung disease. Am J Respir Crit Care Med 2003;167:835–40.

41. Renna M, Schaffner C, Brown K, et al. Azithromycin blocks autophagy and may predispose cystic fibrosis patients to mycobacterial infection. J Clin Invest 2011;121:3554–63.

42. Binder AM, Adjemian J, Olivier KN, et al. Epidemiology of nontuberculous mycobacterial infections and associated chronic macrolide use among persons with cystic fibrosis. Am J Respir Crit Care Med 2013;188:807–12.

43. Catherinot E, Roux AL, Vibet MA, et al, OMA Group. Inhaled therapies, azithromycin and *Mycobacterium abscessus* in cystic fibrosis patients. Eur Respir J 2013;41:1101–6.

44. Radhakrishnan DK, Yau Y, Corey M, et al. Nontuberculous mycobacteria in children with cystic fibrosis: isolation, prevalence, and predictors. Pediatr Pulmonology 2009;44:1100–6.

45. Prevots DR, Adjemian J, Fernandez AG, et al. Environmental risks for nontuberculous mycobacteria. Individual exposures and climatic factors in the cystic fibrosis population. Ann Am Thorac Soc 2014;11:1032–8.

46. Forslow U, Geborek A, Hjelte L, et al. Early chemotherapy for non-tuberculous mycobacterial infections in patients with cystic fibrosis. Acta Paediatr 2003;92:910–5.

47. Leitritz L, Griese M, Roggenkamp A, et al. Prospective study on nontuberculous mycobacteria in patients with and without cystic fibrosis. Med Microbiol Immunol 2004;193:209–17.

48. Martiniano SL, Sontag MK, Daley CL, et al. Clinical significance of a first positive nontuberculous mycobacteria culture in cystic fibrosis. Ann Am Thorac Soc 2014;11:36–44.

49. Martiniano SL, Nick JA. Nontuberculous mycobacterial infections in cystic fibrosis. Clin Chest Med 2015;36:101–15.

50. Whittier S, Olivier K, Gilligan P, et al. Proficiency testing of clinical microbiology laboratories using modified decontamination procedures for detection of nontuberculous mycobacteria in sputum samples from cystic fibrosis patients. The Nontuberculous Mycobacteria in Cystic Fibrosis Study Group. J Clin Microbiol 1997;35:2706–8.

51. Bange FC, Bottger EC. Improved decontamination method for recovering mycobacteria from patients with cystic fibrosis. Eur J Clin Microbiol Infect Dis 2002;21:546–8.

52. Whittier S, Hopfer RL, Knowles MR, et al. Improved recovery of mycobacteria from respiratory secretions of patients with cystic fibrosis. J Clin Microbiol 1993;31:861–4.

53. Steingart KR, Ng V, Henry M, et al. Sputum processing methods to improve the sensitivity of smear microscopy for tuberculosis: a systematic review. Lancet Infect Dis 2006;6:664–74.

54. Brown-Elliott BA, Griffith DE, Wallace RJ Jr. Diagnosis of nontuberculous mycobacterial infections. Clin Lab Med 2002;22:911–25, vi.

55. Buijtels PC, Petit PL. Comparison of NaOH-N-acetyl cysteine and sulfuric acid decontamination methods for recovery of mycobacteria from clinical specimens. J Microbiol Methods 2005;62:83–8.

56. Floto A, ea. Cystic Fibrosis Foundation and European Cystic Fibrosis Society consensus recommendations for the management of nontuberculous mycobacteria in individuals with cystic fibrosis. Thorax, in press.

57. Bange FC, Kirschner P, Bottger EC. Recovery of mycobacteria from patients with cystic fibrosis. J Clin Microbiol 1999;37:3761–3.

58. Ferroni A, Vu-Thien H, Lanotte P, et al. Value of the chlorhexidine decontamination method for recovery of nontuberculous mycobacteria from sputum samples of patients with cystic fibrosis. J Clin Microbiol 2006;44:2237–9.

59. Preece CL, Perry A, Gray B, et al. A novel culture medium for isolation of rapidly-growing mycobacteria from the sputum of patients with cystic fibrosis. J Cyst Fibros 2015. [Epub ahead of print].

60. van Ingen J. Microbiological diagnosis of nontuberculous mycobacterial pulmonary disease. Clin Chest Med 2015;36:43–54.

61. Buchan BW, Riebe KM, Timke M, et al. Comparison of MALDI-TOF MS with HPLC and nucleic acid sequencing for the identification of *Mycobacterium* species in cultures using solid medium and broth. Am J Clin Pathol 2014;141:25–34.

62. CLSI. Susceptibility testing of mycobacteria, nocardia, and other aerobic actinomycetes: approved standard-second edition. CLSI document M24-A2. Wayne (PA): Clinical and Laboratory Standards Institute; 2011.

63. Nash KA, Brown-Elliott BA, Wallace RJ Jr. A novel gene, erm(41), confers inducible macrolide resistance to clinical isolates of *Mycobacterium abscessus* but is absent from *Mycobacterium chelonae*. Antimicrob Agents Chemother 2009;53:1367–76.

64. Doucet-Populaire F, Buriankova K, Weiser J, et al. Natural and acquired macrolide resistance in mycobacteria. Curr Drug Targets Infect Disord 2002;2:355–70.

65. Griffith DE, Brown-Elliott BA, Langsjoen B, et al. Clinical and molecular analysis of macrolide

resistance in *Mycobacterium avium* complex lung disease. Am J Respir Crit Care Med 2006;174: 928–34.

66. Verma N, Spencer D. Disseminated *Mycobacterium gordonae* infection in a child with cystic fibrosis. Pediatr Pulmonology 2012;47:517–8.

67. Mulherin D, Coffey MJ, Halloran DO, et al. Skin reactivity to atypical mycobacteria in cystic fibrosis. Respir Med 1990;84:273–6.

68. Ngan GJ, Ng LM, Jureen R, et al. Development of multiplex PCR assays based on the 16S-23S rRNA internal transcribed spacer for the detection of clinically relevant nontuberculous mycobacteria. Lett Appl Microbiol 2011;52:546–54.

69. Leung KL, Yip CW, Cheung WF, et al. Development of a simple and low-cost real-time PCR method for the identification of commonly encountered mycobacteria in a high throughput laboratory. J Appl Microbiol 2009;107:1433–9.

70. Devine M, Moore JE, Xu J, et al. Detection of mycobacterial DNA from sputum of patients with cystic fibrosis. Ir J Med Sci 2004;173:96–8.

71. Oliver A, Maiz L, Canton R, et al. Nontuberculous mycobacteria in patients with cystic fibrosis. Clin Infect Dis 2001;32:1298–303.

72. Ferroni A, Sermet-Gaudelus I, Le Bourgeois M, et al. Measurement of immunoglobulin G against mycobacterial antigen A60 in patients with cystic fibrosis and lung infection due to *Mycobacterium abscessus*. Clin Infect Dis 2005;40:58–66.

73. Qvist T, Pressler T, Taylor-Robinson D, et al. Serodiagnosis of *Mycobacterium abscessus* complex infection in cystic fibrosis. Eur Respir J 2015; 46(3):707–16.

74. van Ingen J, Egelund EF, Levin A, et al. The pharmacokinetics and pharmacodynamics of pulmonary *Mycobacterium avium* complex disease treatment. Am J Respir Crit Care Med 2012; 186(6):559–65.

75. Clement A, Tamalet A, Leroux E, et al. Long term effects of azithromycin in patients with cystic fibrosis: a double blind, placebo controlled trial. Thorax 2006;61:895–902.

76. Equi A, Balfour-Lynn IM, Bush A, et al. Long term azithromycin in children with cystic fibrosis: a randomised, placebo-controlled crossover trial. Lancet 2002;360:978–84.

77. Saiman L, Marshall BC, Mayer-Hamblett N, et al. Azithromycin in patients with cystic fibrosis chronically infected with *Pseudomonas aeruginosa*: a randomized controlled trial. JAMA 2003;290:1749–56.

78. Wolter J, Seeney S, Bell S, et al. Effect of long term treatment with azithromycin on disease parameters in cystic fibrosis: a randomised trial. Thorax 2002; 57:212–6.

79. Wallace RJ Jr, Brown-Elliott BA, McNulty S, et al. Macrolide/Azalide therapy for nodular/ bronchiectatic *Mycobacterium avium* complex lung disease. Chest 2014;146:276–82.

80. Jeong BH, Jeon K, Park HY, et al. Intermittent antibiotic therapy for nodular bronchiectatic *Mycobacterium avium* complex lung disease. Am J Respir Crit Care Med 2015;191:96–103.

81. Gilljam M, Berning SE, Peloquin CA, et al. Therapeutic drug monitoring in patients with cystic fibrosis and mycobacterial disease. Eur Respir J 1999;14:347–51.

82. Ebert DL, Olivier KN. Nontuberculous mycobacteria in the setting of cystic fibrosis. Clin Chest Med 2002;23:655–63.

83. Cho YJ, Yi H, Chun J, et al. The genome sequence of '*Mycobacterium massiliense*' strain CIP 108297 suggests the independent taxonomic status of the *Mycobacterium abscessus* complex at the subspecies level. PLoS One 2013;8:e81560.

84. Roux AL, Catherinot E, Soismier N, et al, OMA Group. Comparing *Mycobacterium massiliense* and *Mycobacterium abscessus* lung infections in cystic fibrosis patients. J Cyst Fibros 2015;14:63–9.

85. Kearns GL, Trang JM. Introduction to pharmacokinetics: aminoglycosides in cystic fibrosis as a prototype. J Pediatr 1986;108:847–53.

86. de Groot R, Smith AL. Antibiotic pharmacokinetics in cystic fibrosis. Differences and clinical significance. Clin Pharmacokinet 1987;13:228–53.

87. Rey E, Treluyer JM, Pons G. Drug disposition in cystic fibrosis. Clin Pharmacokinet 1998;35: 313–29.

88. Wallace RJ Jr, Brown BA, Griffith DE, et al. Reduced serum levels of clarithromycin in patients treated with multidrug regimens including rifampin or rifabutin for *Mycobacterium avium-M. intracellulare* infection. J Infect Dis 1995;171:747–50.

89. Peloquin CA. Therapeutic drug monitoring in the treatment of tuberculosis. Drugs 2002;62: 2169–83.

90. Moriarty TF, McElnay JC, Elborn JS, et al. Sputum antibiotic concentrations: implications for treatment of cystic fibrosis lung infection. Pediatr Pulmonol 2007;42:1008–17.

91. Jeon K, Kwon OJ, Lee NY, et al. Antibiotic treatment of *Mycobacterium abscessus* lung disease: a retrospective analysis of 65 patients. Am J Respir Crit Care Med 2009;180:896–902.

92. Jarand J, Levin A, Zhang L, et al. Clinical and microbiologic outcomes in patients receiving treatment for *Mycobacterium abscessus* pulmonary disease. Clin Infect Dis 2011;52:565–71.

93. Mitchell JD. Surgical approach to pulmonary nontuberculous mycobacterial infections. Clin Chest Med 2015;36:117–22.

94. Yu JA, Weyant MJ, Mitchell JD. Surgical treatment of atypical mycobacterial infections. Thorac Surg Clin 2012;22:277–85.

95. Jonsson BE, Gilljam M, Lindblad A, et al. Molecular epidemiology of *Mycobacterium abscessus*, with focus on cystic fibrosis. J Clin Microbiol 2007;45: 1497–504.

96. Braun AT, Merlo CA. Cystic fibrosis lung transplantation. Curr Opin Pulm Med 2011;17:467–72.

97. Orens JB, Estenne M, Arcasoy S, et al, Pulmonary Scientific Council of the International Society for Heart and Lung Transplantation. International guidelines for the selection of lung transplant candidates: 2006 update–a consensus report from the Pulmonary Scientific Council of the International Society for Heart and Lung Transplantation. J Heart Lung Transplant 2006;25:745–55.

98. Taylor JL, Palmer SM. *Mycobacterium abscessus* chest wall and pulmonary infection in a cystic fibrosis lung transplant recipient. J Heart Lung Transplant 2006;25:985–8.

99. Zaidi S, Elidemir O, Heinle JS, et al. *Mycobacterium abscessus* in cystic fibrosis lung transplant recipients: report of 2 cases and risk for recurrence. Transpl Infect Dis 2009;11:243–8.

100. Sanguinetti M, Ardito F, Fiscarelli E, et al. Fatal pulmonary infection due to multidrug-resistant *Mycobacterium abscessus* in a patient with cystic fibrosis. J Clin Microbiol 2001;39:816–9.

101. Flume PA, Egan TM, Paradowski LJ, et al. Infectious complications of lung transplantation. Impact of cystic fibrosis. Am J Respir Crit Care Med 1994; 149:1601–7.

102. Gilljam M, Schersten H, Silverborn M, et al. Lung transplantation in patients with cystic fibrosis and *Mycobacterium abscessus* infection. J Cyst Fibros 2010;9:272–6.

103. Lobo LJ, Chang LC, Esther CR Jr, et al. Lung transplant outcomes in cystic fibrosis patients with preoperative *Mycobacterium abscessus* respiratory infections. Clin Transplant 2013;27:523–9.

104. Qvist T, Pressler T, Thomsen VO, et al. Nontuberculous mycobacterial disease is not a contraindication to lung transplantation in patients with cystic fibrosis: a retrospective analysis in a Danish patient population. Transplant Proc 2013; 45:342–5.

105. Watkins RR, Lemonovich TL. Evaluation of infections in the lung transplant patient. Curr Opin Infect Dis 2012;25:193–8.

106. Bange FC, Brown BA, Smaczny C, et al. Lack of transmission of *Mycobacterium abscessus* among patients with cystic fibrosis attending a single clinic. Clin Infect Dis 2001;32:1648–50.

107. Harris KA, Kenna DTD, Blauwendraat C, et al. Molecular fingerprinting of *Mycobacterium abscessus* strains in a cohort of pediatric cystic fibrosis patients. J Clin Microbiol 2012;50:1758–61.

108. Bryant JM, Harris SR, Parkhill J, et al. Whole-genome sequencing to establish relapse or reinfection with *Mycobacterium tuberculosis*: a retrospective observational study. Lancet Respir Med 2013;1:786–92.

109. Aitken ML, Limaye A, Pottinger P, et al. Respiratory outbreak of *Mycobacterium abscessus* subspecies *massiliense* in a lung transplant and cystic fibrosis center. Am J Respir Crit Care Med 2012;185: 231–2.

110. Harris KA, Underwood A, Kenna DT, et al. Whole-genome sequencing and epidemiological analysis do not provide evidence for cross-transmission of *Mycobacterium abscessus* in a cohort of pediatric cystic fibrosis patients. Clin Infect Dis 2015;60: 1007–16.

111. Saiman L, Siegel JD, LiPuma JJ, et al. Infection prevention and control guideline for cystic fibrosis: 2013 update. Infect Control Hosp Epidemiol 2014; 35(Suppl 1):S1–67.

112. Ballarino GJ, Olivier KN, Claypool RJ, et al. Pulmonary nontuberculous mycobacterial infections: antibiotic treatment and associated costs. Respir Med 2009;103:1448–55.

Tuberculosis in Children

Tania A. Thomas, MD, MPH

KEYWORDS

- Tuberculosis • Global epidemiology • Latent infection • Diagnosis • Management • Prevention
- Advocacy

KEY POINTS

- Although tuberculosis (TB) is a preventable condition, it remains a major cause of childhood morbidity and mortality worldwide.
- Young children are at especially high risk of progressing to active TB after exposure.
- Because an accurate diagnostic test for TB in children does not exist, making a confirmatory diagnosis is challenging and requires clinical acumen.
- TB treatment is lengthy, and child-friendly drug formulations are urgently needed.

INTRODUCTION

Despite achieving great public health strides to control tuberculosis (TB) within the United States, it remains an enormous public health issue worldwide. Accurate statistics on pediatric TB cases are difficult to obtain for a multitude of reasons, including under-recognition, challenges in confirming the diagnosis, and under-reporting to national TB programs. The clinical and radiographic manifestations are less specific in children compared with adults and are often confused with bacterial pneumonia. Microbiologic confirmation of disease is limited by the paucibacillary nature of TB in children. In general, TB cultures and newer rapid molecular tests are positive in the minority of children, generally less than 25% to 40% of children with TB disease.[1,2] Additionally, there are often logistic challenges in obtaining adequate specimens from young children. However, in the era of multidrug-resistant TB, in which the organism is resistant to isoniazid and rifampin (the 2 most potent first-line agents), there is an increasing need to attempt culture-confirmation on all children suspected of having TB to inform treatment decisions. Among children who are started on TB therapy, families struggle with proper dose administration due to the lack of pediatric drug formulations and there are programmatic gaps in notifying the national TB programs, leading to under-reporting by the World Health Organization (WHO). Yet, with proper management, including timely treatment initiation with appropriate drug dosages, treatment outcomes are generally favorable.

EPIDEMIOLOGY

The global distribution of childhood TB mirrors that of adults (**Fig. 1**), with a heavy burden of disease in sub-Saharan Africa and Asia.[3] The United States is considered a low-incidence country with less than 4 cases per 100,000 population. Domestically, most TB cases are associated with foreign birth.[4] Between 2008 and 2010, there were 2660 children and adolescents diagnosed with TB.[5] Among them, 31% were foreign born youth. Of the remaining US-born cases, 66% had at least 1 parent who was foreign-born. These trends suggest that most domestic TB cases in children may be exposed in international settings or through foreign-born parents, thus

This article originally appeared in *Pediatric Clinics of North America*, Volume 64, Issue 4, August 2017.
Disclosure Statement: T.A. Thomas reports no financial conflicts of interest. T.A. Thomas is supported by NIH K23 AI097197.
Division of Infectious Diseases and International Health, University of Virginia, PO Box 801340, Charlottesville, VA 22908-1340, USA
E-mail address: tat3x@virginia.edu

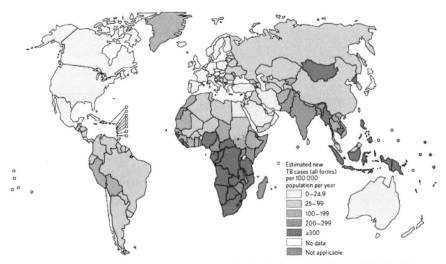

Fig. 1. Estimated TB incidence rates in 2015. (*From* WHO Global Tuberculosis Report 2016; with permission.)

highlighting an opportunity for increased prevention efforts.

Only recently have systematic attempts been made to quantify the disease burden of TB in children on a global scale. In response to increasing attention and demand, the WHO published pediatric-specific disease estimates for the first time in 2012, reporting approximately 500,000 cases of TB among children younger than 15 years of age.[6] However, these were based on extrapolations from adult data, which were heavily weighted on sputum-smear positivity and did not incorporate sufficient adjustments to account for underdetection and under-reporting in pediatric populations.[7] Subsequent modifications to the mathematical models have been incorporated, relying more on transmission dynamics, household demographics, and population-based age structures.[8–10] As a result, the WHO estimates for pediatric TB in the ensuing years doubled: in 2015, the children made up approximately 1 million (10%) of the 10.4 million incident cases.[3] This immense variation in estimated disease burden highlights the challenges in detecting and reporting pediatric TB cases and stresses the importance in resolving these gaps to inform resource allocation and public health efforts.

Similarly, the estimated pediatric mortality burden from TB is poorly quantified. The WHO estimated 210,000 deaths from TB among children in 2015, 24% of whom were coinfected with human immunodeficiency virus (HIV).[3] In many high-burden regions, deaths from TB are often generalized as being due to pneumonia or meningitis. In a recent systematic review from the Child Health Epidemiology Reference Group (CHERG), established by the WHO and the United Nations

Children's Fund (UNICEF), using vital registration and verbal autopsy data, TB was not included as a specific cause of mortality in children younger than 5 years of age.[11] However, it has long been known that TB disproportionately affects young children:

- Mortality from TB is highest among the very young (0–4 years of age) compared with any other age group.[12]
- Infants and young children carry a higher risk of disseminated disease, including TB meningitis and miliary TB, each with associated mortality.[13–15]

The global TB community is working toward "zero TB deaths in children"[16] and meeting this goal relies on coordinated efforts to improve awareness, diagnosis, reporting, and treatment outcomes.

PATHOGENESIS

M tuberculosis complex organisms, which include *M africanum*, *M bovis*, *M bovis* Bacille Calmette-Guerin (BCG), and *M canetti* (and others that do not typically affect humans), are transmitted via the respiratory route when small (1–5 μm) infected droplet nuclei are aerosolized from people with pulmonary or laryngeal TB and inhaled into the alveoli by close contacts.[17] There are many unknown details about the biological events that transpire during early stages of exposure and infection. Alveolar macrophages and dendritic cells are among the first cells to detect and ingest the mycobacteria. Along with additional innate antimicrobial mediators, they trigger a cascade of innate immunologic events to activate complement pathways, stimulate chemokine and proinflammatory cytokine production, including interferon-gamma (IFN-ɣ) and tumor necrosis factor-alpha (TNF-α), and augment opsonization and phagocytosis to clear or control the infection.[18] If this fails or is insufficient, the mycobacteria can invade the lung parenchyma. Adaptive immune responses are triggered when macrophages and dendritic cells present M tuberculosis antigens to T cells, including helper T (Th)-1 type CD4$^+$ T-cells, CD8$^+$ cytotoxic T cells, and gamma-delta (ɣδ) T cells, which further potentiate key cytokine secretion for M tuberculosis control.[19] Historically, B cells were not considered to be an important component in TB immunopathogenesis; however, there is growing evidence to suggest that B cells mediate protection through antigen presentation, cytokine production, and antibody production via interactions with T cells.[20,21] Ultimately, clinicians rely on measuring the T-cell–mediated immune responses as an indication of TB infection, through the IFN-ɣ release assays (IGRAs) and the tuberculin skin test (TST).

Effective immune responses may lead to complete clearance of the pathogen, or containment in a quiescent state. Inadequate or inappropriate immune responses lead to continued replication of the pathogen with progression to pulmonary disease and possible dissemination to extrapulmonary sites. Age and immunologic function are the biggest drivers of progressive disease. Infants and young children have the highest propensity to progress to active, disseminated disease due to the age-related deficiencies and/or downregulation of key immunologic factors (Fig. 2).[22,23] Importantly, the risk of TB disease follows a bimodal pattern. Although children between the ages of 5 to 10 years are at the lowest risk of progressing to disease, adolescents carry higher risks, including reactivation of M tuberculosis

manifesting as active disease after years of successful containment.[5,23]

Additional factors that affect progression of disease include

- Time since exposure, with greatest risk in the first 2 years after exposure
- Mycobacterial burden of exposure
- The virulence of the mycobacterial strain.

Host and environmental risk factors associated with progression include

- Immunocompromising states such as HIV with acquired immune deficiency syndrome (AIDS), malignancy, and chronic renal disease[24,25]
- Socioeconomic conditions such as malnutrition and overcrowding[26,27]
- Environmental exposure to tobacco and indoor air pollutants.[27–29]

NATURAL HISTORY OF DISEASE

TB is often oversimplified as having 2 possible clinical states: latent TB infection (LTBI) or active disease. However, as global targets to end the TB epidemic by 2030 are neared,[30] there is a renewed appreciation for the historically described spectrum of manifestations, including pathogen clearance, dormant states of infection, subclinical disease, nonsevere disease, and severe TB disease[31,32] (Fig. 3). A better understanding of the spectrum of TB may improve resource allocation by focusing treatment and prevention efforts on susceptible individuals, thereby bringing TB control closer.

Immediately after exposure and primary infection from an infectious TB case, there are generally no clinical or radiologic manifestations. It may be possible for humans to clear the pathogen after close contact with infectious sources.[31] Clearance

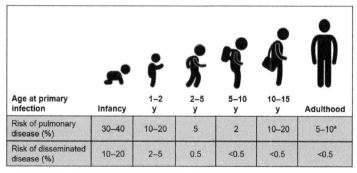

Age at primary infection	Infancy	1–2 y	2–5 y	5–10 y	10–15 y	Adulthood
Risk of pulmonary disease (%)	30–40	10–20	5	2	10–20	5–10[a]
Risk of disseminated disease (%)	10–20	2–5	0.5	<0.5	<0.5	<0.5

Fig. 2. Age-related risks of TB disease after primary infection in the prechemotherapy era.[a] Lifetime risk. (Adapted from Marais BJ, Gie RP, Schaaf HS, et al. The clinical epidemiology of childhood pulmonary tuberculosis: a critical review of literature from the pre-chemotherapy era. Int J Tuberc Lung Dis 2004;8(3):278–85.)

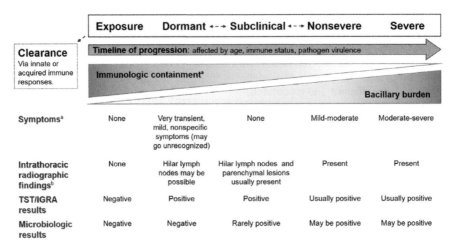

Fig. 3. Spectrum of TB in children. [a] Symptomatology may reflect the intense immunologic reaction to the bacilli, rather than the bacillary burden itself. [b] Findings may not be present if a child has extra-thoracic TB.

of the pathogen may be attributed to genetic resistance to infection or other innate immune responses.[33–36] If clearance occurs through T-cell independent mechanisms, IGRA and TST results should be negative. However, clearance may also occur through T-cell–mediated immunity, which would manifest with positive IGRA and TST results. This latter phenomenon may explain why some people who are diagnosed as having LTBI ultimately have a low likelihood of ever developing active TB disease.[31] However, how often this truly occurs in young children is not well documented.

As per historical description of the timetable of primary TB in children by pediatrician Arvid Wallgren,[37] it takes approximately 4 to 12 weeks after exposure for the adaptive immune responses to reflect evidence of TB infection, as measured by the IGRA and TST. During this period, there is local extension of the infection into the lung parenchyma, termed a Ghon focus, which can manifest clinically with mild, self-limiting, and nonspecific respiratory symptoms, including hypersensitivity reactions such as fevers, erythema nodosum, or phlyctenular conjunctivitis.[23] As demonstrated in contact tracing reports, chest radiographs at this time may also demonstrate transient lymphadenopathy in the hilar and/or mediastinal regions; together with the Ghon focus this is termed a Ghon complex.[38,39] From the regional lymph nodes, the mycobacteria are capable of traversing through the lymphatics into the systemic circulation, allowing for occult hematogenous spread and seeding of distant sites that may serve as a nidus for future disease. Yet, in the absence of effective immunologic control, this stage confers great risk of developing miliary TB and

TB meningitis, although the exact pathogenesis of the latter is still under debate.[40,41] In the approximate 6 months that ensue, intrathoracic lymph node enlargement and/or parenchymal disease may develop; older children may develop pleural effusions. These manifestations can be associated with respiratory and systemic symptoms. In some children, calcifications may develop approximately 1 to 2 years after primary infection; this is associated with a reduced risk of further disease progression.[37,38] However, late manifestations of TB, including reactivation of TB within the lungs or at extrapulmonary sites, do occur.[42]

CLINICAL MANIFESTATIONS OF DISEASE

M tuberculosis is capable of infecting nearly any organ (**Table 1**); however, the most common clinical manifestations of disease are found within the thoracic cavity and peripheral lymph nodes.

Common intrathoracic manifestations include mediastinal or hilar lymphadenopathy and pulmonary parenchymal lesions. Less commonly, the pleura or pericardium become involved. Isolated intrathoracic lymphadenopathy may be detected early after infection and is often not associated with symptoms. However, as these inflammatory reactions progress and lymph nodes enlarge, complications can ensue:

- Small airways may become obstructed or compressed, which may manifest with cough, wheezing, or dyspnea.
- Lymph nodes may caseate or necrose, erupting into the airway, leading to bronchopneumonia and manifesting with cough, dyspnea, malaise, and fever.

Table 1
Extrathoracic manifestation of tuberculosis disease

Organ System	Potential Disease Manifestations
Central nervous system	Meningitis, tuberculoma, stroke
Ocular	Uveitis, phlyctenular conjunctivitis[a]
Otic or nasopharyngeal	Chronic suppurative otitis media, mastoiditis, tonsillitis, laryngeal involvement
Cardiac	Pericardial effusion, secondary right-sided heart failure from extensive pulmonary disease and bronchiectasis
Abdominal	Peritonitis, enteritis, involvement of lymph nodes, visceral involvement (especially liver and spleen)
Genitourinary[b]	Genital involvement possible for females > males, interstitial nephritis, glomerulonephritis
Osteoarticular	Vertebral osteomyelitis, other skeletal involvement possible (especially tubular and flat bones), dactylitis, joint effusions or arthritis (less common), reactive arthritis (Poncet disease)
Lymphatic	Peripheral (cervical > axillary > inguinal region) or central adenopathy
Cutaneous	Numerous manifestations from exogenous infection (chancres, warts) or endogenous spread (lupus vulgaris, pustulonodular lesions), Erythema induratum of Bazin

[a] Hypersensitivity reaction.
[b] Uncommonly seen in young children due to long latency for reactivation in these organs.

- Hypersensitivity reactions may also occur, including pleural effusions, which may provoke symptoms of chest pain, fever, and reduced endurance.

The symptomatology is largely nonspecific and thus can easily be confused with bacterial or viral causes of pneumonia. The classic description of a chronic cough may apply, but it is also important to recognize that young children have a propensity to progress rapidly to disease after exposure. Indeed, TB as a cause of acute pneumonia among young, immunocompromised children is under-recognized.[43] Systematic reviews report *M tuberculosis* as a culture-confirmed pathogen in 7.5% to 12% of children younger than 5 years of age with pneumonia from TB-endemic areas.[43,44] This is a notable finding given the paucibacillary nature of pediatric TB disease.

Extrathoracic manifestations make up approximately 20% to 40% of TB cases, although concomitant overlap with pulmonary disease can occur. The most commonly involved extrathoracic sites are the peripheral lymph nodes or the central nervous system. Lymphadenitis often manifests in the cervical regions with enlarged, painless lymph nodes. Examination typically reveals a solitary rubbery node that lacks erythema or warmth. Over time, adjacent nodes may become palpable and the lesion grows matted and fixed; sinus fistulas may also form. Especially in countries with low TB incidence, other nontuberculous mycobacteria (NTM) are capable of manifesting with lymphadenitis.

Disease within the central nervous system represents the most serious complication of TB, with significant morbidity or mortality occurring in approximately 50% of cases.[45,46] Contributing to the devastating consequences of disease are the subacute onset and nonspecific systemic symptoms during the early stages, such as irritability, fever, and anorexia, and possible focal respiratory or gastrointestinal symptoms. As disease progresses, findings of meningitis become apparent, including vomiting, altered consciousness, convulsions, meningismus, cranial nerve palsies, or signs of raised intracranial pressure. Complications include hydrocephalus, cerebrovascular disease such as stroke and vasculitis, tuberculoma, and coma.[47] Early diagnosis is the key to improved outcomes. However, in the absence of reliable diagnostic tools, a high index of clinical suspicion is required, not only in TB-endemic regions but also in low-TB-burden countries with migrant populations.[48]

DISEASE IN SPECIAL POPULATIONS

Perinatal infection from *M tuberculosis* is thought to be a rare but serious event. It can occur from hematogenous spread of the bacilli from an infected mother through the placenta, which typically results in primary infection of the fetal liver, or directly into the amniotic fluid with subsequent aspiration and infection of the lungs or gastrointestinal tract.[49] TB of the reproductive organs was historically associated with infertility; however, direct extension of TB to the uterus is increasingly being described as a mechanism for congenital TB in the era of improved assistive reproductive technology.[50] Additionally, respiratory transmission may occur postnatally. Symptoms of disease are nonspecific and are indistinguishable from bacterial sepsis or congenital viral infections, and may manifest as early as 2 to 3 weeks of age. A high clinical index of suspicion is required for this relatively uncommon event.

Adolescence represents another uniquely susceptible time for TB progression (see **Fig. 2**). Disease presentation can digress from typical childhood manifestations to include aspects of adult-type TB, including cavitary pulmonary TB or extrathoracic manifestations that are associated with longer incubation periods, such as genitourinary TB.[51] Health care providers should inquire about concurrent substance abuse because this may call for additional counseling or monitoring that is not routinely conducted for younger children. Anxiety and depression may be common, exacerbated by infection control and contact investigation procedures, as well as stigma associated with the diagnosis.[52] These factors, combined with behavioral aspects, add to the vulnerabilities in this population and may lead to poor outcomes, including challenges related to adherence and follow-up.[53,54]

Across the world, HIV infection is the strongest risk factor for TB. Children experience indirect as well as direct effects of HIV. Children who are HIV-uninfected but exposed to others who are HIV-positive also bear an increased risk of TB infection and disease.[55,56] Those who are infected with HIV have impaired cell-mediated immunity to control TB infection, conferring a higher risk of progression to active TB disease after exposure; of reactivation of latent infection; and of severe disease manifestations.[57] Timely recognition of HIV and initiation of antiretroviral therapy (ART) is essential for immune restoration and improved TB control; also important are repeated screening for TB in the early months of ART, as well as provision of isoniazid preventive therapy (in all children who have been ruled out for active TB) and cotrimoxazole therapy.[58–61]

DIAGNOSIS

There are various challenges in confirming the diagnosis of TB in children, which stem from the subtle or nonspecific radiographic findings and the paucibacillary nature of disease.[16,62,63] To date, an accurate diagnostic test for pediatric TB does not exist. Thus, it is essential for clinicians to note that TB is often a clinical diagnosis and, given the poor sensitivity of current diagnostic tools, a negative test does not rule out disease in children.

Confirmatory Tests

A confirmatory diagnosis relies on detecting the pathogen directly; alternative approaches include detecting the histopathologic or host immune response to the pathogen. Direct pathogen-based tests include TB culture, nucleic acid amplification tests (NAATs), and smear microscopy:

- Mycobacterial culture is the gold-standard test for TB, with a limit of detection (LOD) of approximately 10 to 100 colony forming units per milliliter (CFU/mL) in solid or liquid culture media.
  - The sensitivity is generally only 7% to 40% in children due to the paucibacillary nature of disease in this subpopulation.[1,64–66]
  - The time required (up to 6 weeks for positive growth) is sometimes too lengthy to be clinically useful; however, this is a necessary step to conduct phenotypic drug susceptibility testing.
  - When *M tuberculosis* is isolated, it is important to perform drug-sensitivity testing against first-line TB drugs as a start, and against second-line TB drugs as needed.
- Although smear microscopy and NAATs are much faster than culture, these assays are also contingent on the bacillary burden and the sensitivity is even further reduced.[67–71]
  - Smear microscopy has a LOD of approximately 10,000 CFU/mL, conferring limited utility in pediatric TB cases.
  - The newer GeneXpert MTB/RIF (Cepheid, Sunnyvale, California, USA) assay is a NAAT that detects *M tuberculosis* DNA and concomitant resistance to rifampicin with an LOD of 131 CFU/mL.[72] The hands-free and automated nature of this rapid cartridge-based test has contributed to its wide spread implementation throughout high-TB burden settings.[73]
  - GeneXpert only has a pooled sensitivity of approximately 66% compared with TB culture in pediatric populations.[2]
  - Repeated sampling offers incremental yield.[67,68,70]

Of course, collecting a deep respiratory specimen for TB culture from a young child brings added challenges. Most children younger than 7 years do not have the tussive force and/or the oromotor coordination to produce a good-quality expectorated sputum specimen on command. Semi-invasive techniques, such as gastric aspiration and lavage, or sputum induction with or without nasopharyngeal aspiration, may be required. With procedural training, sputum induction provides at least similar microbiologic yield compared with gastric aspiration.[64,65,74] An alternative method of obtaining respiratory specimens includes the use of the string test in which a gelatin capsule containing a nylon string is swallowed and later retrieved for TB culture. The procedure is tolerable for children who can swallow and culture yield seems comparable to sputum induction in preliminary studies.[75,76] Detecting the organism in stool may be an option where GeneXpert MTB/RIF testing is available.[77,78]

In extrapulmonary TB, site-specific specimens for TB culture are often collected, such as cerebrospinal fluid, lymph node aspirates, and other tissue specimens. However, the yield is variable. Mycobacterial blood cultures seem to be of limited yield in children compared with adults.[64,79–81] Histopathologic diagnosis is more commonly pursued in extrapulmonary TB. The overall yield is not well characterized, and depends somewhat on the experience of the proceduralist and pathologist; sensitivity and specificity may be hindered by other granulomatous processes.[82]

Screening Tests

Host immune responses can be harnessed to determine immunologic evidence of exposure to *M tuberculosis*. However, the currently available immunodiagnostics are not able to distinguish between latent infection and active disease. The TST is the oldest screening test for TB and works by measuring a delayed-type hypersensitivity reaction to various mycobacterial antigens within the purified protein derivative. It is well recognized that this test suffers from lack of sensitivity and specificity.[83] To minimize the false-negative and false-positive rates, different cutoffs are used to interpret the findings based on epidemiologic (ie, recent exposure) and individual (ie, host immune response, age) factors.

The newer IGRAs address the issue of specificity cross-reactivity by using particular antigens that are absent from *M bovis* BCG and many other NTM species; this confers a performance advantage among BCG-vaccinated children. Both of the 2 commonly used commercial assays, the T-Spot.TB (Oxford Immunotec, Abingdon, UK) and the QuantiFERON-TB Gold (Qiagen, Hilden,

Germany), require a whole blood sample to measure IFN-γ secretion from CD4$^+$ T cells in response to ex vivo stimulation with RD-1 antigens; neither is preferred over the other.[84] They rely on intact cell-mediated immunity, which may hinder performance in very young children and/or children coinfected with HIV, 2 populations who would benefit most from an accurate diagnostic assay.[85] Advisory bodies have recommended caution when using IGRAs in children younger than 5 years of age due to a lack of data and favor the use of the TST.[86,87] However, increasing experience suggests potential utility in young children, particularly those between 2 to 5 years of age.[84,88]

Overall, when using these screening tests it is helpful to note that

- Each test has inherent limitations leading to false-positives or false-negatives.
- Routine screening should be avoided in favor of targeted testing among children with at least 1 risk factor for TB.
- Neither test can discriminate between latent infection and active disease.
- Among symptomatic children, a negative test (TST or IGRA) never rules out TB disease.[89]

Clearly, improved diagnostics are urgently needed for children.[63] Newer methods that have been evaluated in limited pediatric studies have focused on nonrespiratory specimens, including blood-based assays, such as the T-cell activation marker (TAM) assay, which harnesses host immune responses as a diagnostic biomarker[90]; and transcriptomic studies, which hold promise as a diagnostic and prognostic marker.[91–93] Other biomarkers that have shown promise in adult populations, such as the antibodies in lymphocyte supernatant assay (ALS) and the urinary lipoarabinomannan (LAM) assay, have not shown consistent results in pediatric populations.[94–98] Using feasibly obtained specimens, such as urine, would confer a notable advantage as a point-of-care diagnostic test, and further work in this area is warranted.

Imaging

Given the lack of accurate diagnostic assays, imaging studies serve an important role in the diagnosis of intrathoracic TB. Chest radiographs are the most commonly used method. However, the findings can be relatively nonspecific and interobserver variation may exist, even among experienced clinicians.[99,100] Suggestive findings include

- Intrathoracic lymphadenopathy, for which a lateral film may have additive yield[101]

- Complications such as airway compression
- Air-space disease, which may be indistinguishable from other causes of pneumonia
- Miliary nodules or cavitation (less common).

Computer-aided detection for pulmonary TB has shown initial promise among adults, although performance is reduced in smear-negative (ie, paucibacillary) disease[102]; this technology has not yet been validated among children. Other modalities, such as dose-reduced computed tomography (CT) scans, fluorine-18-fluorodeoxyglucose (FDG)-PET imaging, and MRI, may provide additional detail but are not routinely used in children.

MANAGEMENT

Treatment regimens for pediatric TB have been largely adapted from adults. Because of the slow growth of mycobacteria and the dormant state of many bacilli, the duration of treatment is quite lengthy. Additional considerations include

- Treatment of latent TB requires 3 to 9 months, depending on whether a monotherapy or combination therapy approach is used.
- The short-course regimen for active TB requires 6 months
- More severe forms of TB, including TB meningitis and drug-resistant TB, require 12 or more months of therapy.

Traditional treatment of LTBI typically includes 9-months of isoniazid daily with pyridoxine (for breastfeeding infants, adolescents, and others with low pyridoxine intake). The newer regimen of isoniazid and rifapentine weekly for 12 doses is safe and effective in children 2 to 17 years of age and may improve adherence rates.[103] However, it is currently only available through directly observed therapy (DOT) programs, which may not be routinely available. In attempts to improve completion rates, some experts have increasingly used the 4-month regimen of rifampin, which had typically been recommended for LTBI treatment among those exposed to isoniazid-resistant strains.[104,105]

The standard approach to drug-susceptible TB relies on combination drug therapy with isoniazid, rifampin, pyrazinamide, and ethambutol for the first 2 months, followed by 4 months of isoniazid and rifampin. DOT, typically through a public health department, is recommended to assist with delivery of medications that may be unpalatable, improve adherence, monitor for toxicity, and provide additional support. However, this brings added costs and may not be routinely available.

If drug resistance is confirmed or presumed through an epidemiologic link, treatment should be based on drug susceptibility results (using the index case's results when appropriate). A minimum of 4 active drugs should be used, including an injectable agent. Because of variable efficacy of some second-line drugs, and increased risks of toxicities, treatment decisions should be made in conjunction with a specialist.[86] Close monitoring is required to ensure culture conversion, clinical resolution, and minimize side effects and long-term sequelae.[106]

For the first time in decades, there are newer anti-TB drugs available and in the pipelines. Including children in preclinical and clinical pharmacokinetic studies and efficacy trials is imperative to meeting the goals for global TB control.[107,108] Equally urgent is the need for child-friendly first-line and second-line drugs that are palatable, easily administered, and less toxic.

PREVENTION

TB is a preventable condition that requires coordinated systematic efforts. A child with active TB represents a sentinel event, typically reflecting ongoing transmission in the community. Infection control measures conferring great strides in TB control include household contact investigation of index cases and treatment of LTBI, and these strategies are increasingly being adopted in settings with high TB burden.[30,109] In addition to these public health efforts, primary care providers have an important role in TB control by conducting annual targeted LTBI screening.[86,110]

For decades, the BCG vaccine has been widely used to protect against childhood TB. Although the vaccine is not perfect, it is estimated that 1 year of BCG vaccination prevents over 117,000 deaths per pediatric (<15 years of age) birth cohort.[111,112] However, production issues have led to sizable shortfalls in supply since 2013, which have not completely been resolved. Modeling studies have estimated that the recent shortages may contribute to nearly 20,000 excess childhood deaths from TB.[112]

The development of new and improved TB vaccines is hindered by insufficient understanding of the correlates of protection. As was realized after the modified vaccinia Ankara 85A (MVA85A) TB vaccine trial among human infants, experimental animal models have been unreliable in predicting responses in humans.[113] However, various TB vaccine strategies are under study, including modifications to replace the current BCG, novel vaccines designed to boost responses among BCG recipients, and therapeutic vaccines designed to aid those undergoing TB treatment.[114]

SUMMARY

TB remains a major threat to child health worldwide. Global migration requires that clinicians in low-incidence countries maintain awareness for TB because timely recognition is key, especially in young children. A turning point has been reached in which increased advocacy has stimulated major efforts toward recognition and control of TB in children. However, there is much to be done to meet the ambitious programmatic targets, including widespread uptake of proven prevention efforts and development of newer strategies, including effective vaccines. Dedicated research and development are need for accurate, child-friendly, and fieldable diagnostics. Pediatric-specific studies are necessary to define the best approach to childhood TB using tolerable drugs, especially for drug-resistant TB. All of this requires coordinated efforts and adequate funding. The momentum must continue to end the neglect of childhood TB.

REFERENCES

1. Starke JR. Pediatric tuberculosis: time for a new approach. Tuberculosis (Edinb) 2003;83(1–3): 208–12.
2. World Health Organization. Automated real-time nucleic acid amplification technology for rapid and simultaneous detection of tuberculosis and rifampicin resistance: Xpert MTB/RIF assay for the diagnosis of pulmonary and extrapulmonary TB in adults and children. Policy update. Geneva (Switzerland): World Health Organization; 2013.
3. World Health Organization. Global tuberculosis report 2016. Geneva (Switzerland): World Health Organization; 2016.
4. CDC. Reported Tuberculosis in the United States, 2014. 2015. Available at: http://www.cdc.gov/tb/statistics/reports/2014. Accessed November 30, 2016.
5. Winston CA, Menzies HJ. Pediatric and adolescent tuberculosis in the United States, 2008-2010. Pediatrics 2012;130(6):e1425–32.
6. World Health Organization. Global tuberculosis report 2012 (in IRIS). Geneva (Switzerland): World Health Organization; 2012.
7. Seddon JA, Jenkins HE, Liu L, et al. Counting children with tuberculosis: why numbers matter. Int J Tuberc Lung Dis 2015;19(Suppl 1):9–16.
8. Dodd PJ, Gardiner E, Coghlan R, et al. Burden of childhood tuberculosis in 22 high-burden countries: a mathematical modelling study. Lancet Glob Health 2014;2(8):e453–9.
9. Jenkins HE, Tolman AW, Yuen CM, et al. Incidence of multidrug-resistant tuberculosis disease in children: systematic review and global estimates. Lancet 2014;383(9928):1572–9.
10. World Bank. Population ages 0-14. 2015. Available at: http://data.worldbank.org/indicator/SP.POP.0014.TO.ZS. Accessed November 30, 2016.
11. Liu L, Oza S, Hogan D, et al. Global, regional, and national causes of child mortality in 2000-13, with projections to inform post-2015 priorities: an updated systematic analysis. Lancet 2015; 385(9966):430–40.
12. Frost WH. The age selection of mortality from tuberculosis in successive decades. 1939. Am J Epidemiol 1995;141(1):4–9 [discussion: 3].
13. Karande S, Gupta V, Kulkarni M, et al. Prognostic clinical variables in childhood tuberculous meningitis: an experience from Mumbai, India. Neurol India 2005;53(2):191–5 [discussion: 195–6].
14. van Toorn R, Springer P, Laubscher JA, et al. Value of different staging systems for predicting neurological outcome in childhood tuberculous meningitis. Int J Tuberc Lung Dis 2012;16(5):628–32.
15. Sharma SK, Mohan A, Sharma A, et al. Miliary tuberculosis: new insights into an old disease. Lancet Infect Dis 2005;5(7):415–30.
16. World Health Organization. Roadmap for childhood tuberculosis: towards zero deaths. Geneva (Switzerland): World Health Organization; 2013.
17. Fennelly KP, Martyny JW, Fulton KE, et al. Cough-generated aerosols of Mycobacterium tuberculosis: a new method to study infectiousness. Am J Respir Crit Care Med 2004;169(5):604–9.
18. Basu Roy R, Whittaker E, Kampmann B. Current understanding of the immune response to tuberculosis in children. Curr Opin Infect Dis 2012;25(3): 250–7.
19. Lewinsohn DA, Gennaro ML, Scholvinck L, et al. Tuberculosis immunology in children: diagnostic and therapeutic challenges and opportunities. Int J Tuberc Lung Dis 2004;8(5):658–74.
20. Chan J, Mehta S, Bharrhan S, et al. The role of B cells and humoral immunity in Mycobacterium tuberculosis infection. Semin Immunol 2014;26(6): 588–600.
21. Rao M, Valontini D, Poiret T, et al. B in TB: B cells as mediators of clinically relevant immune responses in tuberculosis. Clin Infect Dis 2015;61(Suppl 3): S225–34.
22. Vanden Driessche K, Persson A, Marais BJ, et al. Immune vulnerability of infants to tuberculosis. Clin Dev Immunol 2013;2013:781320.
23. Marais BJ, Gie RP, Schaaf HS, et al. The clinical epidemiology of childhood pulmonary tuberculosis: a critical review of literature from the prechemotherapy era. Int J Tuberc Lung Dis 2004; 8(3):278–85.

24. Ekim M, Tumer N, Bakkaloglu S. Tuberculosis in children undergoing continuous ambulatory peritoneal dialysis. Pediatr Nephrol 1999;13(7):577–9.

25. Munteanu M, Cucer F, Halitchi C, et al. The TB infection in children with chronic renal diseases [abstract only]. Rev Med Chir Soc Med Nat Iasi 2006;110(2):309–13.

26. Jaganath D, Mupere E. Childhood tuberculosis and malnutrition. J Infect Dis 2012;206(12):1809–15.

27. Chisti MJ, Ahmed T, Shahid AS, et al. Sociodemographic, epidemiological, and clinical risk factors for childhood pulmonary tuberculosis in severely malnourished children presenting with pneumonia: observation in an Urban Hospital in Bangladesh. Glob Pediatr Health 2015;2. 2333794x15594183.

28. Patra S, Sharma S, Behera D. Passive smoking, indoor air pollution and childhood tuberculosis: a case control study. Indian J Tuberc 2012;59(3):151–5.

29. Jafta N, Jeena PM, Barregard L, et al. Childhood tuberculosis and exposure to indoor air pollution: a systematic review and meta-analysis. Int J Tuberc Lung Dis 2015;19(5):596–602.

30. World Health Organization. The end TB strategy. Geneva (Switzerland): World Health Organization; 2015.

31. Dheda K, Schwander SK, Zhu B, et al. The immunology of tuberculosis: from bench to bedside. Respirology 2010;15(3):433–50.

32. Barry CE 3rd, Boshoff HI, Dartois V, et al. The spectrum of latent tuberculosis: rethinking the biology and intervention strategies. Nat Rev Microbiol 2009;7(12):845–55.

33. Cobat A, Gallant CJ, Simkin L, et al. Two loci control tuberculin skin test reactivity in an area hyperendemic for tuberculosis. J Exp Med 2009;206(12):2583–91.

34. Thye T, Owusu-Dabo E, Vannberg FO, et al. Common variants at 11p13 are associated with susceptibility to tuberculosis. Nat Genet 2012;44(3):257–9.

35. Cobat A, Poirier C, Hoal E, et al. Tuberculin skin test negativity is under tight genetic control of chromosomal region 11p14-15 in settings with different tuberculosis endemicities. J Infect Dis 2015;211(2):317–21.

36. Fox GJ, Orlova M, Schurr E. Tuberculosis in newborns: the lessons of the "Lubeck Disaster" (1929-1933). PLoS Pathog 2016;12(1):e1005271.

37. Wallgren A. The time-table of tuberculosis. Tubercle 1948;29(11):245–51.

38. Davies PD. The natural history of tuberculosis in children. A study of child contacts in the Brompton Hospital Child contact clinic from 1930 to 1952. Tubercle 1961;42(Suppl):1–40.

39. Marais BJ, Gie RP, Schaaf HS, et al. A proposed radiological classification of childhood intrathoracic tuberculosis. Pediatr Radiol 2004;34(11):886–94.

40. Donald PR, Schaaf HS, Schoeman JF. Tuberculous meningitis and miliary tuberculosis: the Rich focus revisited. J Infect 2005;50(3):193–5.

41. Janse van Rensburg P, Andronikou S, van Toorn R, et al. Magnetic resonance imaging of miliary tuberculosis of the central nervous system in children with tuberculous meningitis. Pediatr Radiol 2008;38(12):1306–13.

42. Perez-Velez CM, Marais BJ. Tuberculosis in children. N Engl J Med 2012;367(4):348–61.

43. Chisti MJ, Ahmed T, Pietroni MA, et al. Pulmonary tuberculosis in severely-malnourished or HIV-infected children with pneumonia: a review. J Health Popul Nutr 2013;31(3):308–13.

44. Oliwa JN, Karumbi JM, Marais BJ, et al. Tuberculosis as a cause or comorbidity of childhood pneumonia in tuberculosis-endemic areas: a systematic review. Lancet Respir Med 2015;3(3):235–43.

45. Chiang SS, Khan FA, Milstein MB, et al. Treatment outcomes of childhood tuberculous meningitis: a systematic review and meta-analysis. Lancet Infect Dis 2014;14(10):947–57.

46. Bang ND, Caws M, Truc TT, et al. Clinical presentations, diagnosis, mortality and prognostic markers of tuberculous meningitis in Vietnamese children: a prospective descriptive study. BMC Infect Dis 2016;16(1):573.

47. van Toorn R, Solomons R. Update on the diagnosis and management of tuberculous meningitis in children. Semin Pediatr Neurol 2014;21(1):12–8.

48. van Well GT, Paes BF, Terwee CB, et al. Twenty years of pediatric tuberculous meningitis: a retrospective cohort study in the western cape of South Africa. Pediatrics 2009;123(1):e1–8.

49. Peng W, Yang J, Liu E. Analysis of 170 cases of congenital TB reported in the literature between 1946 and 2009. Pediatr Pulmonol 2011;46(12):1215–24.

50. Flibotte JJ, Lee GE, Buser GL, et al. Infertility, in vitro fertilization and congenital tuberculosis. J Perinatol 2013;33(7):565–8.

51. Cruz AT, Hwang KM, Birnbaum GD, et al. Adolescents with tuberculosis: a review of 145 cases. Pediatr Infect Dis J 2013;32(9):937–41.

52. Franck C, Seddon JA, Hesseling AC, et al. Assessing the impact of multidrug-resistant tuberculosis in children: an exploratory qualitative study. BMC Infect Dis 2014;14:426.

53. Blok N, van den Boom M, Erkens C, et al. Variation in policy and practice of adolescent tuberculosis management in the WHO European Region. Eur Respir J 2016;48:943–6.

54. Enane LA, Lowenthal ED, Arscott-Mills T, et al. Loss to follow-up among adolescents with tuberculosis

in Gaborone, Botswana. Int J Tuberc Lung Dis 2016;20(10):1320–5.

55. Marquez C, Chamie G, Achan J, et al. Tuberculosis infection in early childhood and the association with HIV-exposure in HIV-uninfected children in rural Uganda. Pediatr Infect Dis J 2016;35(5):524–9.

56. Cotton MF, Slogrove A, Rabie H. Infections in HIV-exposed uninfected children with focus on sub-Saharan Africa. Pediatr Infect Dis J 2014;33(10):1085–6.

57. Verhagen LM, Warris A, van Soolingen D, et al. Human immunodeficiency virus and tuberculosis co-infection in children: challenges in diagnosis and treatment. Pediatr Infect Dis J 2010;29(10):e63–70.

58. Anigilaje EA, Aderibigbe SA, Adeoti AO, et al. Tuberculosis, before and after antiretroviral therapy among HIV-infected children in Nigeria: what are the risk factors? PLoS One 2016;11(5):e0156177.

59. Zar HJ, Cotton MF, Strauss S, et al. Effect of isoniazid prophylaxis on mortality and incidence of tuberculosis in children with HIV: randomised controlled trial. BMJ 2007;334(7585):136.

60. Bwakura-Dangarembizi M, Kendall L, Bakeera-Kitaka S, et al. A randomized trial of prolonged co-trimoxazole in HIV-infected children in Africa. N Engl J Med 2014;370(1):41–53.

61. Crook AM, Turkova A, Musiime V, et al. Tuberculosis incidence is high in HIV-infected African children but is reduced by co-trimoxazole and time on antiretroviral therapy. BMC Med 2016;14:50.

62. Cuevas LE, Petrucci R, Swaminathan S. Tuberculosis diagnostics for children in high-burden countries: what is available and what is needed. Paediatr Int Child Health 2012;32(Suppl 2):S30–7.

63. Nicol MP, Gnanashanmugam D, Browning R, et al. A blueprint to address research gaps in the development of biomarkers for pediatric tuberculosis. Clin Infect Dis 2015;61(Suppl 3):S164–72.

64. Thomas TA, Heysell SK, Moodley P, et al. Intensified specimen collection to improve tuberculosis diagnosis in children from Rural South Africa, an observational study. BMC Infect Dis 2014;14:11.

65. Zar H, Hanslo D, Apolles P, et al. Induced sputum versus gastric lavage for microbiological confirmation of pulmonary tuberculosis in infants and young children: a prospective study. Lancet 2005;365(9454):130–4.

66. Nicol MP, Zar HJ. New specimens and laboratory diagnostics for childhood pulmonary TB: progress and prospects. Paediatr Respir Rev 2011;12(1):16–21.

67. Nicol MP, Workman L, Isaacs W, et al. Accuracy of the Xpert MTB/RIF test for the diagnosis of pulmonary tuberculosis in children admitted to hospital in Cape Town, South Africa: a descriptive study. Lancet Infect Dis 2011;11(11):819–24.

68. Zar HJ, Workman L, Isaacs W, et al. Rapid molecular diagnosis of pulmonary tuberculosis in children using nasopharyngeal specimens. Clin Infect Dis 2012;55(8):1088–95.

69. Rachow A, Clowes P, Saathoff E, et al. Increased and expedited case detection by Xpert MTB/RIF assay in childhood tuberculosis: a prospective cohort study. Clin Infect Dis 2012;54(10):1388–96.

70. Zar HJ, Workman L, Isaacs W, et al. Rapid diagnosis of pulmonary tuberculosis in African children in a primary care setting by use of Xpert MTB/RIF on respiratory specimens: a prospective study. Lancet Glob Health 2013;1(2):e97–104.

71. Detjen AK, DiNardo AR, Leyden J, et al. Xpert MTB/RIF assay for the diagnosis of pulmonary tuberculosis in children: a systematic review and meta-analysis. Lancet Respir Med 2015;3(6):451–61.

72. Helb D, Jones M, Story E, et al. Rapid detection of *Mycobacterium tuberculosis* and rifampin resistance by use of on-demand, near-patient technology. J Clin Microbiol 2010;48(1):229–37.

73. Lawn SD, Nicol MP. Xpert(R) MTB/RIF assay: development, evaluation and implementation of a new rapid molecular diagnostic for tuberculosis and rifampicin resistance. Future Microbiol 2011;6(9):1067–82.

74. Hatherill M, Hawkridge T, Zar HJ, et al. Induced sputum or gastric lavage for community-based diagnosis of childhood pulmonary tuberculosis? Arch Dis Child 2009;94(3):195–201.

75. Chow F, Espiritu N, Gilman RH, et al. La cuerda dulce–a tolerability and acceptability study of a novel approach to specimen collection for diagnosis of paediatric pulmonary tuberculosis. BMC Infect Dis 2006;6:67.

76. Nansumba M, Kumbakumba E, Orikiriza P, et al. Detection yield and tolerability of string test for diagnosis of childhood intrathoracic tuberculosis. Pediatr Infect Dis J 2016;35(2):146–51.

77. Marcy O, Ung V, Goyet S, et al. Performance of Xpert MTB/RIF and alternative specimen collection methods for the diagnosis of tuberculosis in HIV-infected children. Clin Infect Dis 2016;62(9):1161–8.

78. Banada PP, Naidoo U, Deshpande S, et al. A novel sample processing method for rapid detection of tuberculosis in the stool of pediatric patients using the Xpert MTB/RIF assay. PLoS One 2016;11(3):e0151980.

79. Pavlinac PB, Lokken EM, Walson JL, et al. *Mycobacterium tuberculosis* bacteremia in adults and children: a systematic review and meta-analysis. Int J Tuberc Lung Dis 2016;20(7):895–902.

80. Heysell SK, Thomas TA, Gandhi NR, et al. Blood cultures for the diagnosis of multidrug-resistant and extensively drug-resistant tuberculosis

among HIV-infected patients from rural South Africa: a cross-sectional study. BMC Infect Dis 2010;10:344.

81. Gray KD, Cunningham CK, Clifton DC, et al. Prevalence of mycobacteremia among HIV-infected infants and children in northern Tanzania. Pediatr Infect Dis J 2013;32(7):754–6.

82. Fukunaga H, Murakami T, Gondo T, et al. Sensitivity of acid-fast staining for *Mycobacterium tuberculosis* in formalin-fixed tissue. Am J Respir Crit Care Med 2002;166(7):994–7.

83. Dunn JJ, Starke JR, Revell PA. Laboratory diagnosis of *Mycobacterium tuberculosis* infection and disease in children. J Clin Microbiol 2016; 54(6):1434–41.

84. Starke JR, Byington CL, Maldonado YA, et al. Interferon-γ release assays for diagnosis of tuberculosis infection and disease in children. Pediatrics 2014;134(6):e1763–73.

85. Mandalakas AM, Detjen AK, Hesseling AC, et al. Interferon-gamma release assays and childhood tuberculosis: systematic review and meta-analysis. Int J Tuberc Lung Dis 2011;15(8):1018–32.

86. American Academy of Pediatrics. Tuberculosis. In: Kimberlin D, Brady M, Jackson M, et al, editors. Pediatrics. 30th edition. Elk Grove Village (IL): American Academy of Pediatrics; 2015. p. 805–31.

87. Lewinsohn DM, Leonard MK, LoBue PA, et al. Official American Thoracic Society/Infectious Diseases Society of America/Centers for Disease Control and Prevention Clinical Practice Guidelines: Diagnosis of Tuberculosis in Adults and Children. Clin Infect Dis 2017;64(2):111–5.

88. Grinsdale JA, Islam S, Tran OC, et al. Interferon-gamma release assays and pediatric public health tuberculosis screening: the San Francisco program experience 2005 to 2008. J Pediatr Infect Dis Soc 2016;5(2):122–30.

89. Starke JR. Interferon-gamma release assays for the diagnosis of tuberculosis infection in children. J Pediatr 2012;161(4):581–2.

90. Portevin D, Moukambi F, Clowes P, et al. Assessment of the novel T-cell activation marker-tuberculosis assay for diagnosis of active tuberculosis in children: a prospective proof-of-concept study. Lancet Infect Dis 2014;14(10):931–8.

91. Anderson ST, Kaforou M, Brent AJ, et al. Diagnosis of childhood tuberculosis and host RNA expression in Africa. N Engl J Med 2014;370(18):1712–23.

92. Zak DE, Penn-Nicholson A, Scriba TJ, et al. A blood RNA signature for tuberculosis disease risk: a prospective cohort study. Lancet 2016; 387(10035):2312–22.

93. Zhou M, Yu G, Yang X, et al. Circulating microRNAs as biomarkers for the early diagnosis of childhood tuberculosis infection. Mol Med Rep 2016;13: 4620–6.

94. Rekha RS, Kamal SM, Andersen P, et al. Validation of the ALS assay in adult patients with culture confirmed pulmonary tuberculosis. PLoS One 2011;6(1):e16425.

95. Thomas T, Brighenti S, Andersson J, et al. A new potential biomarker for childhood tuberculosis. Thorax 2011;66(8):727–9.

96. Chisti MJ, Salam MA, Raqib R, et al. Validity of antibodies in lymphocyte supernatant in diagnosing tuberculosis in severely malnourished children presenting with pneumonia. PLoS One 2015;10(5): e0126863.

97. Blok N, Visser DH, Solomons R, et al. Lipoarabinomannan enzyme-linked immunosorbent assay for early diagnosis of childhood tuberculous meningitis. Int J Tuberc Lung Dis 2014;18(2):205–10.

98. Nicol MP, Allen V, Workman L, et al. Urine lipoarabinomannan testing for diagnosis of pulmonary tuberculosis in children: a prospective study. Lancet Glob Health 2014;2(5):e278–84.

99. Du Toit G, Swingler G, Iloni K. Observer variation in detecting lymphadenopathy on chest radiography. Int J Tuberc Lung Dis 2002;6(9):814–7.

100. Swingler GH, du Toit G, Andronikou S, et al. Diagnostic accuracy of chest radiography in detecting mediastinal lymphadenopathy in suspected pulmonary tuberculosis. Arch Dis Child 2005;90(11): 1153–6.

101. Smuts NA, Beyers N, Gie RP, et al. Value of the lateral chest radiograph in tuberculosis in children. Pediatr Radiol 1994;24(7):478–80.

102. Breuninger M, van Ginneken B, Philipsen RH, et al. Diagnostic accuracy of computer-aided detection of pulmonary tuberculosis in chest radiographs: a validation study from sub-Saharan Africa. PLoS One 2014;9(9):e106381.

103. Villarino ME, Scott NA, Weis SE, et al. Treatment for preventing tuberculosis in children and adolescents: a randomized clinical trial of a 3-month, 12-dose regimen of a combination of rifapentine and isoniazid. JAMA Pediatr 2015; 169(3):247–55.

104. Cruz AT, Starke JR. Safety and completion of a 4-month course of rifampicin for latent tuberculous infection in children. Int J Tuberc Lung Dis 2014; 18(9):1057–61.

105. Cruz AT, Martinez BJ. Childhood tuberculosis in the United States: shifting the focus to prevention. Int J Tuberc Lung Dis 2015;19(Suppl 1):50–3.

106. Seddon JA, Furin JJ, Gale M, et al. Caring for children with drug-resistant tuberculosis: practice-based recommendations. Am J Respir Crit Care Med 2012;186(10):953–64.

107. Nachman S, Ahmed A, Amanullah F, et al. Towards early inclusion of children in tuberculosis drugs trials: a consensus statement. Lancet Infect Dis 2015;15(6):711–20.

108. Srivastava S, Deshpande D, Pasipanodya JG, et al. A combination regimen design program based on pharmacodynamic target setting for childhood tuberculosis: design rules for the playground. Clin Infect Dis 2016;63(Suppl 3): S75-9.

109. Morrison J, Pai M, Hopewell PC. Tuberculosis and latent tuberculosis infection in close contacts of people with pulmonary tuberculosis in low-income and middle-income countries: a systematic review and meta-analysis. Lancet Infect Dis 2008;8(6): 359-68.

110. van der Heijden YF, Heerman WJ, McFadden S, et al. Missed opportunities for tuberculosis screening in primary care. J Pediatr 2015;166(5): 1240-5.e1.

111. Mangtani P, Abubakar I, Ariti C, et al. Protection by BCG vaccine against tuberculosis: a systematic review of randomized controlled trials. Clin Infect Dis 2014;58(4):470-80.

112. Harris RC, Dodd PJ, White RG. The potential impact of BCG vaccine supply shortages on global paediatric tuberculosis mortality. BMC Med 2016; 14(1):138.

113. Tameris MD, Hatherill M, Landry BS, et al. Safety and efficacy of MVA85A, a new tuberculosis vaccine, in infants previously vaccinated with BCG: a randomised, placebo-controlled phase 2b trial. Lancet 2013;381(9871):1021-8.

114. Principi N, Esposito S. The present and future of tuberculosis vaccinations. Tuberculosis (Edinb) 2015;95(1):6-13.

Moving?

Make sure your subscription moves with you!

To notify us of your new address, find your **Clinics Account Number** (located on your mailing label above your name), and contact customer service at:

Email: journalscustomerservice-usa@elsevier.com

800-654-2452 (subscribers in the U.S. & Canada)
314-447-8871 (subscribers outside of the U.S. & Canada)

Fax number: 314-447-8029

Elsevier Health Sciences Division
Subscription Customer Service
3251 Riverport Lane
Maryland Heights, MO 63043

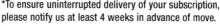
*To ensure uninterrupted delivery of your subscription, please notify us at least 4 weeks in advance of move.

ELSEVIER

Printed and bound by CPI Group (UK) Ltd, Croydon, CR0 4YY

08/05/2025

01864743-0004